*An Introduction to
Immunology*

An Introduction to Immunology

Edited by

**E. M. Lance
P. B. Medawar
E. Simpson**

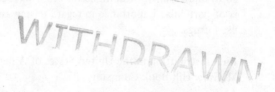

McGraw-Hill Book Company
A Blakiston Publication

*New York   St. Louis   San Francisco   Auckland
Bogotá   Düsseldorf   Johannesburg   London   Madrid
Mexico   Montreal   New Delhi   Panama   Paris
São Paulo   Singapore   Sydney   Tokyo   Toronto*

First published 1977
© 1977 by Peter Medawar

Wildwood House Ltd, 29 King Street, London WC2

NOTICE

Medicine is an ever-changing science. As new research and clinical experience broaden our knowledge, changes in treatment and drug therapy are required. The editors and the publisher of this work have made every effort to ensure that the drug dosage schedules herein are accurate and in accordance with the standards accepted at the time of publication. Readers are advised, however, to check the product information sheet included in the package of each drug they plan to administer to be certain that changes have not been made in the recommended dose or in the contraindications for administration. This recommendation is of particular importance in regard to new or infrequently used drugs.

First distribution in the United States of America by McGraw-Hill Book Company 1977

Library of Congress Cataloging in Publication Data
(Library of Congress Catalog Number)
77-2160
ISBN 0-07-036108-8

Printed and bound in Great Britain by
Biddles Ltd, Guildford, Surrey

Contents

An Introduction to Immunology

lymphoid tissue; diffuse gut associated lymphoid tissue; lymphatic circulation; lymphocytes: differentiation in the thymus; differentiation in the periphery; B cells. Antigen recognition: interaction with antigen; interactions between lymphoid cells: synergy; T-B synergy; antergy; T-B antergy. Lymphocyte kinetics; alterations in kinetics after immunization. Other lymphoid cells; macrophages; non-specificity of inflammation.

Contents

Foreword

Several excellent elementary texts on immunology are already on the market, and this little
book is not intended to add yet another to
their number, for it is in no sense a micro-
textbook, but a series of – as we hope –read-
able essays which will be most useful if they
are read straight through. Moreover, we are
addressing a rather special audience. Many
introductory texts, though they may seem
easy to their authors, are quite hard going for
people who have very little background of
thought in immunology, or whose knowledge
of immunology dates back to the days when
its subject matter was thought to be coextensive with the actions and interactions of
antigens and antibodies. This book is intended
for busy medical practitioners, physicians and
surgeons, for students of biology or 'paramedical' sciences who want the kind of
introductory text that will empower them to
read or anyhow to refer to modern immuno-

logical papers without blank incomprehension. Although the orientation throughout is not primarily clinical, special attention has naturally been paid to clinical implications in the chapters on transplantation (Chapter 3), on tumour immunity (Chapter 4), and of course in the chapter on immunological diseases (Chapter 5).

The lengths of the several chapters are not proportional to the importance of the subjects they deal with, but rather to the amount of explanation that is needed in order to provide an adequate introduction to the literature. Detailed references have not been given, since that is not the purpose of the text, but it may be said that a natural book to turn to next would be Humphrey and White's *Immunology for Students of Medicine*, 3rd revised edition (Blackwell Scientific Publications, Oxford, 1970). With very rare exceptions – all of a kind most immunologists would understand and approve of – we have omitted all proper names and personal attributions of the discoveries and ideas of immunology, believing that immunologists who might have hoped and expected to enjoy the spectacle of their names in print will be equally gratified to think that their work has been 'received' into a text as elementary as this. The omission of any detailed treatment of blood groups and of erythrocyte antigens generally was deliberate, for the subject is not one of great intrinsic difficulty and is specially well served by admirable elementary textbooks, such as Race and Sanger, *Blood Groups in Man*, 5th edition (Blackwell Scientific Publications, Oxford, 1968). The shortcomings of the chapter on transplantation biology can be remedied by reference to Billingham and Silvers, *The Immunology of Transplantation* (Prentice-Hall Inc., New Jersey, 1971).

It has not been taken for granted that our readers will have had a medical or paramedical training to first degree level, and therefore some very elementary ground has been gone over, particularly in relation to lymph and lymphatics. This is because zoologists (for example) are normally kept in ignorance of the existence of a lymphoid system. Being among the 'soft parts' of an animal, it has left behind it no fossil record which could be used as testimony of evolution, and had therefore very little to interest comparative anatomists of an older school.

The chapters are short, for we had it in mind that many readers would wish to read the book straight through at a sitting. The Introduction provides a general overview of immunology and the remaining chapters deal in greater detail with those aspects of immunology which are specially prominent today.

The authors have not been nervously on their guard against repetitions or overlaps; on the contrary, some repetition may well be thought helpful.

In one way or another all members of the staff of the Surgical Sciences Division and Transplantation Biology section of the MRC Clinical Research Centre, Watford Road, Harrow, have taken part in the preparation of this book: Dr E. M. Lance, Sir Peter Medawar, Dr Valerie Jones, Dr Stella Knight, Dr Elizabeth Simpson, Dr D. J. Pinto, Mrs Ruth Hunt, Mrs Joy Heys, Mrs Valerie Price.

The authors of the more technical chapters are distinguished by initials to acquit them of any guilt for the errors of fact or judgement made elsewhere. Persons who take offence at being told what they already know, e.g. about the nature and use of logarithms (p. 23), are reading the wrong book.

Medical Research Council E.M.L. ⎞
Clinical Research Centre P.B.M. ⎬ Editors
Watford Road E.S. ⎠
Harrow
Middlesex HA1 3UJ

Introduction

In the past five or ten years immunology has grown more rapidly than any other branch of biomedical science. There are several reasons for this. Immunology is a subject of great intrinsic interest which has thrown light on protein synthesis, the molecular basis of specificity, information transfer in biological systems and cellular behaviour generally. In addition it is directly relevant to tissue transplantation (Chapter 3) and to the etiology and cure of disease, including malignant disease (Chapter 4).

The word 'immunity' has a technical meaning that does not correspond exactly with its everyday usage. Some animals contract and recover from infectious diseases as a result of a specific adaptive response known as an 'immunological response'; other animals may not contract the disease in the first place because they are not susceptible to it. Human beings develop immunity to the measles virus, but are not susceptible to distemper. Dogs are not susceptible to measles. An organism may be non-susceptible for many reasons, one being that it does not provide a suitable culture medium for the infectious agent; thus the rodent malarial organism *Plasmodium berghei* does not proliferate in newborn rats because of an insufficiency of the essential growth factor *p-aminobenzoic acid.*

Antigens, immunogens, immunogenicity. Substances that arouse an immunological response are said to be *antigenic.* Whole organisms can be said to be antigenic but it is not very helpful or informative to describe them as 'antigens' because it is desirable wherever possible to specify the part of the antigenic agent considered as a whole which excites and is primarily the target of the immune response. With tissue cells and erythrocytes this will often be the cell surface, in bacteria the cell wall, and in viruses the protein capsule.

Qualifications for antigenicity. Members of all classes of chemical compounds (including some which have not yet been synthesized and of which no organism can therefore ever have had experience) may be antigenic, but even so the power to excite an immune response usually resides in only part of the molecule – *the determinant group.*

Haptens, adjuvants, adjuvanticity. Molecules which are not antigenic in themselves but which nevertheless confer specific reac-

2

tivity upon some larger molecule of which they may form a part are referred to as *haptens*. Large molecular size is no longer thought to be a necessary qualification for antigenicity, for many haptens have molecular weights of the order of only hundreds. Nevertheless, in order to act as such an antigenic molecule must have the power to engage with and if necessary to recruit reactive cells from the responding organism (see Chapter 2). This property is often referred to as 'adjuvanticity'. Adjuvanticity may or may not be an intrinsic property of the molecule, but some otherwise non-antigenic substances can be made to be so merely by physical incorporation into adjuvants. The most famous is Freund's adjuvant, a stiff water-in-oil emulsion made with the help of surface-active agents and (in 'complete' Freund adjuvant) also containing dead mycobacteria. A property all antigens have in common is 'foreignness' to the immunological reaction system.

Specificity. Much of the biological interest of immunological reactions and much of their usefulness in throwing light upon information transfer and protein synthesis turns on their specificity, i.e. the unique one-to-one pairing of stimulus and response. Non-specificity always requires some special explanation or excusatory comment. If the reaction against antigen A extends in some measure to antigen B this will often be because A and B are closely related chemical structures – a property which has been put to use for taxonomic purposes (as in Nuttall's famous studies of blood relationships). Though it should be added that zoologists seldom accept serological evidence of affinity unless it sustains their own preconceptions.

Immunogens as a subclass of antigens. Antigens are usually administered in such a way as to arouse immunity in one or other of its many forms (see below). They may also be administered at such a dosage or in such a form, or by such a route or at such an age that they arouse not immunity but 'tolerance' (Chapter 3). Tolerance is a state of specific non-reactivity towards a substance that would otherwise arouse an immune response. The word 'antigen' is now used to refer to agents that can excite either immunity or tolerance, the former capability being distinguished by the use of the word *immunogen*. Sometimes the only difference between an immunogen and an antigen which induces tolerance is the possession or lack of intrinsic adjuvanticity (see above).

Information and information flow. The figurative use of the word 'information' - borrowed from communications engineering - is now common in all branches of biology, including immunology. *Information* refers to order or orderliness or to some particularly relevant aspect of it. Anything which exemplifies or embodies structural orderliness of the same specificity - e.g. a programme or a set of instructions for the assembly of a specific structure or for a particular physiological or behavioural performance – may be said to carry or embody the same information. It is a fundamental principle of biology, exemplified by all systems which have been critically examined, that at a molecular level information can flow in one direction only: from nucleic acid to protein or other macromolecule and never from protein to protein. Antibodies are proteins (Chapter 1) but a protein or carbohydrate antigen cannot inform the synthesis of an antibody, i.e. cannot confer upon it, by reason of its own structure, the specific complementary structure appropriate to an antibody. Thus no matter what the modality of the immune response, an immunogen can only awaken some pre-existing potentiality encoded in the nucleic acid of the responding cell.

The New Immunology was the term used by Macfarlane Burnet, one of its main founders, to refer to the immunology that grew up in the 1950s in awareness of the dogma on information flow that has just been propounded. Microbiologists who had confronted a cognate problem in the study of microbial genetics, especially bacterial adaptation, also played an important part in founding the new immunology by insisting that immunological reactions must necessarily have selective or Darwinian character as opposed to an 'instructive' or Lamarckian character. A crucially important paper, by Jerne, in the new immunology was indeed entitled 'The Natural Selection Theory of Antibody Formation'. The theory that prevailed until then that a cell might somehow be 'taught' by antigen how to make an antibody – has obvious Lamarckian parallels.

Modalities of the immune response. Notwithstanding the miscarriages and maladaptations referred to in Chapters 3 and 5, the effect of an immune response is generally to kill, immobilize, make harmless, sequester or otherwise inactivate the antigen or its vehicle. The adaptive value of immunological responses was first made very clear by the existence of those immunological deficiency diseases (Chapter 5) in the most extreme of which – agammaglobulinaemia – the victim is unable to synthesize proteins of the class to which antibodies belong (Chapters 1 and 5). Agammaglobulinaemic patients can be kept alive only by antibiotics.

The chief manifestations of the immune response will be summarized very briefly now and dealt with more fully later. Neither here nor in the paragraphs that follow can the account be exhaustive because not all modalities of the immune response have yet been discovered.

Humoral immunity. The term 'humoral immunity' does not refer to some revival of the old doctrine of humours (bile, choler, phlegm, etc.) but to the fact that many immunological reactions, particularly those directed against micro-organisms, are mediated through the action of circulating blood proteins known as 'antibodies' (Chapter 1). Antibodies are soluble blood proteins modified in such a way that their structure is complementary to that of the determinant group of the antigen (see above).

Humoral immunity was at one time taken to be coextensive with all immunity, but over the past ten or fifteen years it has become increasingly clear that an entirely new category must be recognized, namely *cell mediated immunity (CMI)*, which may or may not be (but usually is) accompanied by humoral antibody formation. In CMI the principal effector or agent is not a soluble protein in the bloodstream, but an immuno-logically activated lymphoid cell – one which has been modified by exposure to antigen in such a way as to empower it or its progeny to engage with the antigen or its vehicle (Chapter 2). The cell mediated immunities include so-called 'delayed type hypersensitivity' as in the tuberculin reaction; transplantation immunity (Chapter 3); tumour immunity (Chapter 4) and some forms of autoimmunity (Chapter 5).

In addition to CMI in a conventional sense, it is almost certainly necessary to recognize yet another variant of the immune response having some of the qualities of both humoral immunity and CMI: the existence of cell-dependent antibodies which exercise their action only after attachment to a circulating cell, the identity of which is not certainly known.

Blood groups; 'natural antibodies'. Familiar blood group reactions, such as the agglutination of the erythrocytes of someone of group A by serum from someone of group B or Group 0, are invariably regarded as immunological. Thus A and B blood group substances are orthodox antigens belonging to the class of nitrogen-containing polysaccharides known as mucoids and present on the red cell surface. Disregarding the very many finer subdivisions of antigens, the distribution of antigens and antibodies follows the following well-known pattern:

Antigens:	A	B	AB	0
Antibodies:	anti-B	anti-A	nil	anti-A
				anti-B

What is unusual about this situation is that the antibodies corresponding to each antigen are ostensibly ready-made. Each individual has antibodies to the antigen that is lacking. Antibodies of this kind are sometimes called 'natural' with the implication that they do not arise in response to an antigenic stimulus but are naturally preformed. The tendency nowadays, however, is to believe that all antibodies are formed by active response to an antigenic stimulus, in this case not by the erythrocyte antigens themselves but by closely related antigens that are known to be present in some micro-organisms. The 'natural' antibodies against the erythrocytes of very distant species found in the blood of rabbits or human beings can have arisen in no other way.

The antibodies corresponding to antigens M, N and the Rh series are not found 'naturally' but are formed in response to antigenic provocation. The Rh antigens were discovered by testing upon human erythrocytes the antibodies formed by the injection of the blood of *rhesus* monkeys into rabbits.

Miscarriages of immunity. Although immunological reactions generally are beneficial and indeed essential for life, some are sufficiently deleterious to justify the recognition of 'immunological diseases' (Chapter 5). Allergies such as asthma and urticaria are self-evidently deleterious; so are the misadventures that lead to blood transfusion accidents and to the rejection of foreign grafts (Chapter 3). These latter reactions may be regarded as the price paid for the existence of a reaction system very highly attuned to the discernment and elimination of 'non-self' substances. Indeed, the acceptance of a transplanted foreign skin graft may be regarded teleonomically as a disease of which its rejection is the cure. Both blood transfusion and tissue transplantation are wholly artificial acts so perhaps it is not surprising that they do not enjoy any dispensation from the effects of immune reactivity.

Sensitivity, hypersensitivity. The injection of antigen into the skin of an immunized human being, guinea pig or rabbit will often give rise to a violent inflammatory response which is prompt in onset (when humoral immunity is involved) or delayed for a matter of hours or even a day or two if the immunity is cell mediated. It was at one time common practice to describe all cell mediated immunities generically as 'delayed type hypersensitivity reactions' and in guinea pigs and human beings all CMI, including the transplant rejection process, may indeed be made to manifest itself as a delayed cutaneous inflammatory response. Nevertheless any such nomenclature should be frowned upon because it is clearly inadvisable to name a whole class of reactions by reference to one inconstant and comparatively trivial manifestation. Many laboratory animals such as rats and mice do not show the characteristic delayed skin reddening that accompanies CMI in guinea pigs and man. They do, however, manifest the local lymphocytic infiltration which is the true distinguishing mark of CMI. In human beings hypnotic suggestion can be used to eliminate the visible reddening that accompanies a delayed type skin reaction, but as it cannot eliminate the cellular element of the reaction, there is no likelihood of its being used to prolong the life of foreign transplants. Rabbits, guinea pigs and human beings are also susceptible to a violent form of immediate cutaneous reactivity known as the *Arthus* reaction. Because CMI is so often accompanied by humoral antibody formation, skin reactions are often compounded of the immediate and delayed types and differentiation between the two elements is a difficult and usually an expert matter. Other forms of sensitivity in humoral systems are dealt with later (refer particularly to IgE in Chapters 1 and 5).

Cells engaged in immunological reactivity (detailed treatment, Chapter 2). It was at one time quite usual to describe as an 'immunologically competent cell' a cell qualified to undertake immunological reactions, but now that the nature and extent of cellular co-operation, additive activity, synergy and antergy are more widely understood the term is dropping out of use. Apart from their function as effector cells in CMI and as antibody formers as in humoral immunity, the activities performed by cells in the immune response include antigenic recognition, engagement with and processing of antigen and information transfer (e.g. from macrophage to lymphocyte and perhaps from lymphocyte to lymphocyte).

Blood leucocytes. Polymorphs, the most numerous white blood cells, are not known to play a *specific* part in immunological reactions; their great importance as effector cells is to phagocytose particulate antigenic matter, particularly when the antigens have been coated with antibody. *Monocytes* are also phagocytic and there is evidence that they may 'process' antigen and make it available to *lymphocytes* which are themselves non-phagocytic, but which are both the recognition cells and the effector cells of CMI.

Lymph, lymphatics, lymphocytes (see Chapter 2). The blood supply of the tissues is both afferent and efferent, but the *lymphatics* are exclusively efferent. The vague use by physiologists of the word 'lymph' to refer to tissue fluid generally is mistaken. Lymph is the fluid content of the special vessels known as lymphatics. The composition of lymph is closely similar to that of the blood plasma from which it derives and with which it is in equilibrium. Antigens introduced into the body parenterally (i.e. otherwise than by mouth) usually reach immunological reaction centres through lymphatics. This also applies to intraperitoneal injection and to intracutaneous injection ('all intradermal injections are in reality intralymphatic' – McMaster). Lymphocytes are the characteristic cellular element of lymphatics and like the lymph in which they are contained, they eventually pour into the blood stream. Lymphocytes are a heterogeneous population but an important proportion is now known to circulate and recirculate through blood and lymph. It was at one time taken for granted that lymphocytes were very short-lived cells and 'Where do lymphocytes go?' was a question repeatedly asked of experimental pathologists by people aware that vast numbers (of the order of 10^{10} or 10^{11}) enter the blood stream daily through the thoracic duct – an unaccountable phenomenon in the days when it was thought that all such lymphocytes were newly formed. Studies on the occurrence of chromosomal abnormalities in the lymphocytes of patients who had received intensive therapeutic radiation many years previously show that small lymphocytes may have lifetimes of the order of years and even ten years is not an unheard-of figure.

B cells and T cells; the thymus. Lymphoid cells engaged in immunological responses may be divided into two major categories: B cells and T cells. Experiments carried out on developing chicks *in ovo* have shown that embryos deprived surgically or hormonally of the so-called *Bursa of Fabricius* hatch into chicks which, though capable of CMI, do not synthesize immunoglobulins or, therefore, antibodies. This deficiency is presumed to be due to the absence of a cell which depends on the *bursa* (hence 'B cell') for its origin or maturation. The term B cell is also used in the context of mammalian immunology to refer to a cell homologous with the bursa-dependent cell of chicks. Experiments using cell transfer have shown that bone marrow is a source of such cells in mammals. The term T cell is used to refer to a cell dependent upon the thymus gland for its origin or maturation. The function of the mammalian thymus was almost totally obscure until immunobiologists showed by experiments on newborn mice and observations on human beings that in the absence of the thymus the faculty of CMI does not develop. Moreover the thymus performs a continuing function in later life, for in the absence of the thymus an irradiated adult mouse will not fully recover CMI.

Thymus-dependent or thymus-derived cells are the principal recirculating moiety of the lymphocyte population. During the course of circulation thymus-derived cells congregate temporarily in the paracortical or 'thymus-dependent' areas of lymph nodes (Chapter 2). These lymphocytes, moreover, are distinguished by the presence of a characteristic tissue-specific antigen, *theta*, so that an anti-theta antibody can be used to remove T cells from a mixed population. Thymus-derived cells also react to so-called plant lectins such as phytohaemagglutinin (PHA) and pokeweed mitogen (PWM) by 'transformation', i.e. by swelling up, synthesizing DNA, and ultimately dividing. This transformation can also be brought about by the action of antibodies directed against lymphocytes and by soluble antigens to which the lymphocytes are sensitive; thus a certain proportion of lymphocytes from a tuberculin positive subject will transform in the presence of tuberculin.

Lymph nodes. On its way to the blood stream all lymph percolates through one or more sets of lymph nodes, the functional architecture of which is described in Chapter 2. Lymph nodes are not lymphocyte factories but stations along their pathway of circulation.

Humoral immunity: antibodies. Humoral immunity is the form of immunity of which the effectors are circulating immunoglobulins (Chapter 1). Two examples may be cited: the response aroused by the injection into a rabbit of sheep red blood cells (SRBC) – say 10^8 cells in 1 ml suspending fluid given intravenously – or the response excited by the intravenous or subcutaneous injection of 1 ml 1% bovine serum albumin into a rabbit.

The response aroused by a *first* exposure to SRBC – the 'primary response' – is of the scale and tempo illustrated by Fig. 1. After this first exposure the rabbit remains for some weeks in a specially reactive condition, such that a *second* injection of a similar or even a much lesser quantity of antigen excites a quicker and stronger response – the 'secondary response' – also shown in Fig. 1.

The form taken by an antigen-antibody reaction *in vitro* depends upon the physical state of the antigen and on the way in which the antigen and antibody confront each other. In the response to SRBC the forms of interaction most commonly used for the identification and measurement of antibodies are agglutination and lysis. In the agglutination reaction SRBC are exposed in agglutination

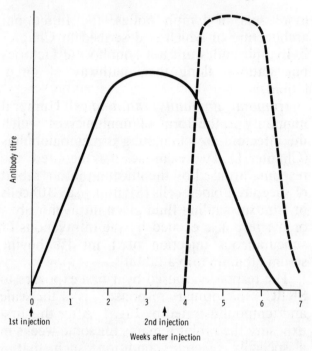

Fig. 1. Diagram illustrating the differences of tempo and amplitude between primary and secondary humoral antibody responses (see text).
Solid line shows a primary response seen to reach a peak about three weeks after antigen injection.
Dotted line shows secondary response, much prompter in onset and reaching a higher peak value.

tubes or other suitable reaction cells to falling dilutions of the antiserum, each dilution usually one half the concentration of the one before. By convention the 'titre' of the serum is the *reciprocal* (e.g. 64, 128) of the highest dilution (e.g. 1/64, 1/128) at which agglutination can be discerned. When lysis is to be

16

investigated, the reaction mixture will consist of three, not just of two parts. These are (1) SRBC, (2) antiserum in falling dilutions, (3) fresh serum as a source of complement.* Lysis is in effect the rupture of cell membranes by complement and the liberation of cell contents into the surrounding medium, which in the lysis of red cells therefore becomes pink. The endpoint is often assessed by eye as for agglutination reactions, but a much more exact variant of the lysis technique is to label the target cells with a radioactive marker so that the degree of lysis can be measured in terms of the fraction of total radioactivity liberated into the supernatant fluid, after non-lysed cells have been removed by centrifugation. It goes without saying that the serum used as the source of complement should not cause lysis of SRBC on its own account.

In order that concentrations of complement should be made uniform and that agglutination reactions should not be confounded by haemolysis at high concentrations of antibody-containing serum it is customary to 'inactivate' a serum that has to be titrated for agglutinins or lysins by heating it to 56 °C for 25 minutes to destroy complement.

The reaction excited by the injection of a

---

* *Complement*. The general name for a complex system of factors in normal fresh blood serum that brings about the lysis of antigenic cells in the presence of specific antibody. Complement is destroyed by heating an antiserum to 56°C for 20–30 minutes – a procedure to which antibodies are resistant.

soluble protein may be made to manifest itself *in vitro* in a variety of different ways. The simplest reaction is one in which the antibody-containing serum is simply mixed with an antigen solution, whereupon, if the ratio of reagents has been well chosen, a precipitate will form and may be recognized by the turbidity of the mixture. This precipitation reaction is very sensitive to variations of antigen and antibody concentrations, and for this reason a slightly more sophisticated variant is to layer antigen and antibody one on top of the other, having at the bottom, of course, the fluid of higher specific gravity. Set up in this way – the 'ring test' – a positive tube is marked by the formation of a ring of precipitate at the interface between antigen and antibody. For qualitative analysis a more sophisticated way of causing this reaction to occur is to allow one reagent to diffuse into the other entrapped in a gelatin or other suitable gel. Alternatively the gel may be prepared in such a way that both antigen and antibody diffuse towards each other from separate reservoirs in the medium. The advantage of this procedure is that antigen and antibody confront each other over a very wide range of concentrations, of which one is likely to be optimal, so that a precipitate will form and be easily visible.

Exact quantitative work on the estimation of antibody is, however, no longer allowed to depend upon what must necessarily be a somewhat subjective and non-scalar assessment of the presence or absence of precipitation lines, or of pinkness in a supernatant fluid. The tendency rather is to measure that basic property of an antibody upon which all its other manifestations depend, i.e. its capacity to bind with antigen. If a soluble protein antigen (BSA for example) is radioactively labelled, it can be caused to interact with anti BSA antibody over a very wide range of concentrations. The antibody can then be precipitated by adding an equal volume of saturated ammonium sulphate solution to the reaction mixture, whereupon the washed antibody precipitate, entraining any antigen to which it has been bound, may be centrifuged down, washed and counted for radioactivity.

Another, quite different method of assessing the intensity of a humoral immune response is to take advantage of the fact that an immunized animal disposes of antigen much more quickly than an animal which has had no experience of that antigen before. If an antigen such as BSA is introduced into the blood stream of a rabbit it will disappear through ordinary metabolic processes at a rate proportional to its concentration at any one time. This pattern of decay (in the simple case exponential) is such that the logarithm of the concentration or antigen in the blood stream forms a straight line when plotted against time. In an animal that has already been immunized by the same antigen, however, the rate of decay is more-than-exponential, for specific immunological processes are now added to the ordinary metabolic removal of the foreign protein from the blood stream. This accelerated rate of decay is most easily assessed by introducing into the blood stream antigen which has been radioactively labelled, though not of course by methods so drastic as to expedite its removal on that account alone. This procedure is often used in practice to distinguish between normal reactivity and specific non-reactivity ('tolerance'). In tolerant animals the rate of decay of antigen is simply exponential whereas in the animal which is, or becomes, immunized, decay is faster, as explained above. To illustrate the importance of the physical form of antigen and antibody in determining the kind of reaction that occurs when they confront each other, it may be pointed out that precipitin reactions towards soluble antigens may often be converted into agglutination reactions – by, for example, coating with antigen particles or cells which do not otherwise participate in the reaction: when collodion particles or SRBC previously treated with tannic acid are coated with the antigen, exposure to antibody will usually cause agglutination, so the precipitin can be read as an agglutinin. It is for reasons such as these that antibodies are not now referred to as 'precipitins', 'lysins' or 'agglutinins' as if these were category differences, instead of merely signifying different and variable manifestations of reactivity.

Immunoelectrophoresis. This is the name given to a gel diffusion method which combines the discriminating power of diffusion with that of electrophoresis: a gel diffusion reaction is caused to take place in an electrical field so that the reagents are spread out as with ordinary electrophoresis in accordance with the electrical charges they bear. Of all the methods of qualitative analysis used in immunology, immunoelectrophoresis has the highest resolving power.

Absorption, complement fixation. Antibodies are of course used up in specific immunological reactions, and this property makes it possible to remove them from a serum in which their presence would be a nuisance – e.g. from a guinea pig serum which is to be used as a source of complement in a reaction turning upon lysis. The procedure is of course pointless unless the guinea pig serum contains so-called 'natural' antibodies directed against the target cells that are to undergo lysis. In such a situation the guinea pig serum is mixed under ice cold conditions with well-washed target cells so that antibody-absorption can take place without contamination of the serum by lysis. The serum is recovered by centrifugation, whereupon the process may be repeated for a second or if necessary a third time until the serum will cause no lysis of the target cells except in the presence of an antibody directed specifically against them. As a separate consideration, antigen-antibody reactions usually involve the using up of complement – 'complement fixation' – a property that is quite widely used for identifying an interaction between antigen and antibody when no more direct means is available. The Wasserman test for syphilis is a case in point.

Table 1   Illustrating the relationship between halving dilutions of antibody, antibody titres and logs to the base 2

Dilutions	1/2	1/4	1/8	1/16	1/32	1/64	1/128	....
Titre	2	4	8	16	32	64	128	256....
Titre as power of 2	1	2	3	4	5	6	7	8.....
Log (base 2)	1	2	3	4	5	6	7	8.....

Table 2   As Table 1, but illustrating the corresponding situation when each dilution is one-third the strength of its predecessor

Dilutions	1/3	1/9	1/27	1/81	1/243	1/729	1/2187
Titre	3	9	27	81	243	729	2187
Titre as power of 3	1	2	3	4	5	6	7
Log (base 3)	1	2	3	4	5	6	7

Use of logarithms to express titres. A series of halving dilutions of antibody corresponds to a series of titres – the reciprocals of the dilutions – which necessarily form a series of powers of 2 (see Table 1). For this reason the titres are sometimes expressed as logarithms to the base 2. The use of logs to the base 2 is useful only when halving dilutions are used. If however each dilution were one-third of the concentration of its predecessor in the series, then logarithms to the base 3 would be more appropriate (Table 2).

Toxins and antitoxins. Among the most important and therapeutically useful of the functions of antibodies is their power to neutralize bacterial exotoxins – metabolic products liberated by bacteria which are among the most poisonous substances known; indeed, second only to puffer fish venom, the exotoxin of *Clostridium botulinum* is the most poisonous natural substance known: a few microlitres of a culture of *Cl. botulinum* can kill a guinea pig, and a few milligrams can kill a human being. Diphtheria toxin produces a destructive inflammatory lesion at a point of intracutaneous injection. This property is made the basis of the 'Schick' test of immune status with respect to diphtheria. A quantity of toxin only just sufficient to raise the visible inflammatory spot is injected into one arm and the same quantity of heated toxin into the other arm to act as a control. If antidiphtheric antibodies are present there will be no reddening. Reddening at the site of injection of the active toxin signifies a toxin still active, and therefore an absence of immunity. (This then works the opposite way round to the tuberculin reaction: in the Mantoux test inflammation signifies *sensitivity* to tubercular antigens whereas in the Schick test inflammation signifies the lack of diphtheria antitoxin.)

Reagins and hypersensitivity reactions. Mention has already been made of 'delayed type' hypersensitivity reactions as cutaneous manifestations of cell mediated immunity and therefore of 'sensitivity', such as sensitivity to tubercle bacilli and other mycobacteria. Two quite different skin reactions are associated with humoral immunity. The immediate 'wheal and flare' type of reaction is provoked by the intracutaneous injection of antigens that arouse allergy in some individuals, e.g. pollen antigens or penicillin. The antibodies responsible for these local manifestations of allergy are sometimes referred to as 'reaginic' or as reagins (Chapter 1). As a separate consideration some animals, notably rabbits, are specially susceptible to a violent and sometimes necrotizing inflammatory reaction when an antigen and the corresponding humoral antibody meet in the skin: this is the 'Arthus' reaction which is described as direct when antigen is introduced into the skin of an actively immunized subject and passive when immunity has been passively conferred by a blood or serum transfer. A 'reversed passive' skin reaction occurs when antigen is introduced systemically and antibody is injected locally. The Arthus reaction is sometimes referred to as a 'local anaphylaxis'. Systemic anaphylaxis leading to shock and perhaps death occurs in, for example, immunized human beings or guinea pigs when antigen is injected systemically into an antibody-containing subject. In extreme cases anaphylaxis is marked by respiratory distress, rapid shallow breathing, an accelerated heart beat, widespread oedema and even death.

An allergic manifestation of special importance, because of its experimental uses, is the Schultz-Dale reaction: uterine muscle or strips of ileum from a sensitized guinea pig contract *in vitro* when exposed to low concentration of the antigen responsible for sensitization. Much research has been devoted to identifying the pharmacological effectors (notably histamine) through which the Schultz-Dale reaction is mediated. The reaction is still a very useful tool to pharmacologists, but is no longer the subject of very active investigation by immunologists.

Reaginic antibodies belong to the immunoglobulin class E (Chapter 1).

Transfer of humoral immunity. Immune states for which humoral antibodies are responsible can be transferred from one animal to another of the same species by transfusions of serum or blood. Transfer from one species to another is complicated by the fact that the sera are themselves antigenic and can thus cause undesirable immunity reactions on their own account. For this reason the prophylactic use of antisera raised in distantly foreign species – e.g. anti-tetanus serum raised in horses – is slowly being supplanted by the practice of active immunization using heat-killed or formalin-treated organisms or inactivated toxins (toxoids). Nevertheless the use of human immunoglobulin concentrates has served a very useful purpose and an antiserum raised in distantly related species may still be used in emergencies. The subject's reaction to such an antiserum will depend upon the number of exposures he may previously have had to the same foreign serum.

Humoral immunity acquired at second hand by serum transfer etc. is referred to as 'passive' immunity. One of the most important forms of passive immunity is that which protects newborn mammals and birds. In birds immunity is transferred from mother to young predominantly through the yolk of the egg. In mammals the routes of passive immunization vary from species to species: intrauterine transfer is often mainly through the yolk sac, and to some degree also through the placenta. In general, however, the most important source of antibodies is the milk, particularly the first milk (colostrum) at the stage when the gut of the newborn is still permeable by antibodies.

Transfer of cell mediated immunity; 'trans-

fer factor'. The most obvious operational difference between humoral immunity and CMI is that whereas the former can be transferred from one animal to another by transfusions of antibody-containing blood or serum, the latter can be transferred only by the inoculation of lymph node fragments or, preferably, by transfusions of dissociated lymphoid cells from sensitized donors. The recipients of these sensitized cells acquire at second hand the immune state characteristic of their donors.* Lymphoid cells must be alive if they are to transfer immunity: heating them to 47°C for 15–20 minutes abolishes their power to do so. The obligatory use of living cells has imposed a grave handicap on both experimental and clinical uses of transference of CMI, because on the face of it it restricts transference to a host organism so closely related genetically to the cell donor that transferred cells will not be rejected as allografts (Chapter 3).

A new episode of research began when students of hypersensitivity in human beings disregarded the fact that living cells intended to transfer tuberculin sensitivity would certainly be executed by an allograft reaction and showed that tuberculin sensitivity could nevertheless in fact be transferred from one human being to another by injections of living

* Immunity passively acquired by cell transfer is said to be 'adoptive' in origin.

leucocytes from the buffy coat of the sensitive donor's blood.

It was next thought a natural step to kill the cells before transfer – and this was done by alternately freezing and thawing them and breaking up the sticky nucleoprotein tangles inevitably so formed by the addition of trace quantities of deoxyribonuclease (DNAase). Very surprisingly, this disrupted and DNAase treated extract also transferred sensitivity. Later experiments showed that the active agent within the material transferred, named 'transfer factor' by H. S. Lawrence, would pass through a dialysis membrane, and had a molecular weight of the order of thousands.

For very many years experimentation on transfer factor was confined to human volunteers. Progress was inevitably very slow and for that reason has been severely criticized by experimentalists with indefinitely large numbers of inbred mice at their command. Nevertheless a number of painstaking and laborious experiments point to the specificity of the action of transfer factor – a property which, though reassuring from an immunological point of view, nevertheless raises some doubts about whether so small a molecule would be informational in function, as its specificity seems to require, and critics of transfer factor have not forgotten that molecules distantly akin to those of the class to which transfer factor was thought to belong – e.g. synthetic double stranded polyribonucleotides – are non-specific immuno-potentiating agents (Chapter 4).

The potential clinical use of transfer factor is for the reinstatement of specific immune deficiencies (Chapter 5) and rather striking clinical successes have been recorded in the treatment of generalized mucocutaneous candidiasis, but much yet remains to be discovered: the cell from which transfer factor originates, the cell to which it attaches itself upon transfer, and its mode of action generally.

Transfer factor is not known to have a natural function in the immune response, but one possibility is that it is the agent by means of which a regional immunological reaction is scaled up from purely regional to systemic dimensions (see also p. 55).

Antibodies. All antibodies are immunoglobulins and there is some reason to believe that all immunoglobulins are antibodies, i.e. that all serum globulins of the sizes and structural characteristics described in Chapter 1 have some antibody specificity, so that perhaps there are no 'neutral' or nonsense immunoglobulins which are not antibodies to anything, and which have only the general physiological function of, for example, helping to regulate the colloid osmotic pressure of the serum.

Allotypes. Quite apart from the differentiation of antibodies into the classes described in Chapter 1, and from the fact that the polypeptide chains from which they are composed have both a variable and a constant part, the immunoglobulins, like most other macromolecules in the body also exhibit 'polymorphism', i.e. exist in a variety of structurally distinct forms ('allotypes') with a characteristic partition in the population. As with polymorphism of other kinds, it is presumed that allotypy is maintained by the action of selective forces (in this case of a quite unknown character). At all events, the frequency of even the least frequent variant is greater than can be accounted for by the pressure of recurrent mutation. The structural traits that distinguish different allotypes in immunoglobulin molecules are present on both light and heavy chains. Allotype differences are inherited in simple Mendelian style.

Recognition of antigen. The first episode in an immunological reaction must necessarily be the recognition of antigen. According to the dogma on information flow described on p. 4 the capacity to recognize and respond in some specific way to an antigen must be ready-made in the reacting system. In effect this can only mean that 'antigen-sensitive' cells responsible for the detection of antigen must exist in variant forms numerous enough to match any antigen with which the organism may be confronted. Antibody molecules have both variable and constant parts and the different capabilities of responding to antigen must clearly reside in the variable part. It is known moreover that some B lymphocytes –

presumably those specifically responsible for antigen recognition – carry on their surfaces trace quantities of immunoglobulin which equip them to recognize antigen. There are still conflicting views about the origin of antibody variants. In one view, the zygote contains all information necessary to underwrite the formation of all the varieties of antibody needed to recognize the antigens which the organism is likely to be confronted with during life. If this interpretation is correct, an antigen acts in a way essentially analogous to that of an embryonic 'inducer', i.e. it completes the differentiation of a lymphoid cell into a clone enjoying one specific and restricted capability, in this case that of reacting in some way upon a specific antigen. In an alternative view, information comes into being during the animal's own development – and necessarily by 'mutation', for mutation is defined as the inception of new heritable information. The two processes are not incompatible, of course, for a randomizing process might be superimposed upon whatever programmes are embodied in the zygote itself. The recognition of antigen is dealt with more fully in Chapter 2.

P.B.M.

CHAPTER ONE
Classes of Immunoglobulin

An immunoglobulin molecule is built up from four polypeptide chains: two identical light chains (LL) and two identical heavy chains (HH) united by disulphide (S-S) bridges. The immunoglobulin molecules to be found in a single individual belong to five classes, G, M, A, D and E. The classification is based on distinctive amino acid sequences within the constant regions of the heavy chains (Fig. 2a).

The members of these different immunoglobulin classes have special functions which must be to some extent determined by these structural differences. For example, only some classes of antibody can combine with complement and this combining site is in the so-called hinge region of the constant part of the heavy chain (Fig. 2a).

Light chains also have a constant region in which differences of structure divide them into two types, kappa (κ) and lambda (λ). Differences in light chain structure have not so

Classes of Immunoglobulin

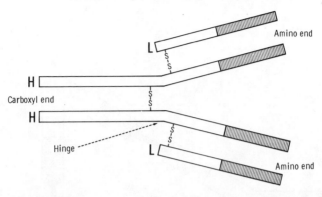

Fig. 2a. Illustrating the molecular skeleton of an immunoglobulin molecule.
LL – Light chains.
HH – Heavy chains.
S-S – Disulphide bonds.
The constant region is unshaded, the variable region indicated by vertical hatchings.

far been correlated with functional differences between immunoglobulin molecules.

Antibodies with both types of L chain are found in all immunoglobulin classes A-E.

At the opposite end of the immunoglobulin molecule (the amino end) is the variable (V) region – that which is responsible for recognizing and combining with antigen. Both the heavy and light chains of an antibody are thus important in the recognition of antigen (Fig. 2b).

The most abundant immunoglobulin class, *IgG*, (still sometimes referred to as 7S gamma globulin because of its properties on sedimen-

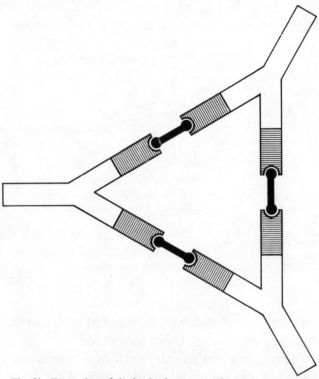

Fig. 2b. Formation of the lattice between antigen and antibody by showing how the Y-shaped skeleton is opened out in the union with antigen (indicated by dark, dumbell shaped unions between the variable regions of antibody molecules).

tation in the ultracentrifuge) forms about 80% of the immunoglobulin of a normal human being and has a molecular weight of about 150,000. IgG can traverse the placenta. In man and some other species it is thus responsible for all the immunity which the fetus acquires passively by the placental route (see p. 26). Monocytes (macrophages) have receptors for

IgG; IgG antibody can bind to micro-organisms to form a complex which is then readily engulfed by these macrophages. Most IgG molecules also combine with complement. These biological functions make IgG a principal defence against infection.

IgM (19S) antibodies are distinctive because of their high molecular weight, about 950,000. They are pentamers consisting of five molecules, each of four polypeptide chains. For this reason each IgM antibody has many more antibody combining sites than an IgG molecule and is specially effective in agglutination and in sensitizing cells for lysis by complement. The formation of IgM antibodies is an early response to many antigens, followed later by IgG.

IgA is the class of antibody responsible for the protection of epithelial (mucous) surfaces such as those of the gut and buccal mucosa: in dimeric form it is abundant in saliva, tears and lung and gut secretions and in colostrum which provides the main immunological protection of the suckling.

IgD has no distinctive biological activity and indeed has only recently been shown to function as an antibody.

By far the smallest amount of immunoglobulin in the body is contributed by IgE but IgE has a distinctive biological activity which identifies it easily. IgE antibodies can fix upon the surface of mast cells of their own species for long periods, and when antigen combines with them a series of events is triggered off which leads to the release of vasoactive amines from the mast cells and thus for the symptoms of anaphylaxis and allergy (see p. 114).

The properties of the principal immunoglobulins are listed in Table 3.

V.J.

Classes of Immunoglobulin

Table 3 Summary of the Properties of the Principal Immunoglobulins

Class	Polymeric State	Molecular Weight	Sedimentation coefficient	Percent of total immunoglobulin	Power to fix complement	Biological properties
IgG	Monomer	150,000	7S	75	+	Traverses the placenta; enhances phagocytosis of micro-organisms.
IgM	Pentamer	950,000	19S	10	+	Early response to infection; efficient in agglutination and cytolysis.
IgA	Monomer, dimer and tetramer	160,000	7–11S	14	−	Major immunoglobulin at mucous surfaces and in secretions.
IgD	Monomer	185,000	7S	1	−	Found on the surface of blood lymphocytes with IgM.
IgE	Monomer	190,000	8S	0.003	−	High concentrations induced by helminth infections. Causes allergic symptoms.

CHAPTER TWO
Lymphocytes and the Lymphatic System

Anatomy

The cells which collectively form the immunological response system of the organism are
housed in a system of lymphoid organs and
lymphoid aggregates, the entire system being
served by traffic channels that ensure
communication with all parts of the body.
Lymphoid organs may be classified functionally into generative and service units. The
former, i.e. the 'central lymphoid tissue',
consists of the thymus and the *Bursa of Fabricius.*

The thymus, a paired organ in the media-
stinum, is responsible for the maturation of
those cells whose functions include the transaction of cell mediated immunity and 'help'
for antibody production. Within the connec-
tive tissue stroma of the thymus are numerous
tightly-packed small lymphoid cells: 'thymocytes'. In addition there are cords of epithelial

cells whose detailed function is unknown; they are presumed to govern the maturation and differentiation of thymocytes. It may well be that these cells are responsible for the elaboration of a thymic hormone, thymosin.

The *Bursa of Fabricius*, found only in birds, arises in close association with the intestinal tract near the junction of the large and small bowel. The bursa is required for the development of the cells engaged in humoral immunity and, as with the thymus, is marked by the specially close association between epithelial and lymphoid cells. It is widely assumed that mammals possess an organ homologous with the bursa; but none has yet been identified with certainty.

Peripheral lymphoid organs include the lymph nodes and the spleen. *Lymph nodes* occur singly or in chains and are widely distributed throughout the body. They are so positioned that they lie on the lymphatic pathway draining every major organ and appendage, and every body cavity with the exception of the anterior chamber of the eye and the intra-cranial cavity. They are named by their location: mesenteric, brachial, axillary, etc., and all have a very similar architecture (Fig. 3). In the resting lymph node the afferent lymphatic vessel empties into a peripheral sinus beneath which is a cortex composed of a few layers of small lymphocytes. Beneath the cortex the paracortex consists of loose aggregations of small lymphocytes aggregated around small blood vessels and finally the medulla consists of a series of sinusoids draining into the efferent lymphoid channel. The sinusoids are lined by cells of the phagocytic and lymphoid series.

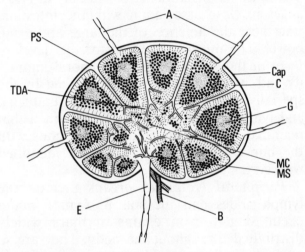

Fig. 3. Illustrating the general architecture of a lymph node as described in the text.
C, capsule.
G, germinal centre.
B, blood vessels.
MC, medullary cords.
MS, medullary sinus.
Notice that afferent lymphatics (A) enter the convexity of the node, and that efferent lymphatics (E) emerge from the hilum of the node.

A lymph node undergoing an active immune response is very different. The whole organ becomes swollen and hyperplastic and the cortex now contains numerous ball-like clusters of lymphoid cells and macrophages which are referred to as *germinal centres.* The paracortex comes to be densely packed with lymphoid cells many of which are in mitosis and blast transformation – cells whose cytoplasm now stains brilliantly with pyronin. In addition, adjacent to blood vessels lymphoid sinuses which were previously not visible are now seen to be crowded by aggregates of small lymphocytes. The medulla, depending upon how long the reaction has been sustained, may become transformed into sheets and plates of plasma cells. After withdrawal of the immunizing stimulus there is a gradual reversion to the resting pattern.

The spleen, a very complex organ, is divided into red and white pulp. The red pulp, concerned largely with haematological activity, will not be considered here. The white pulp is scattered diffusely throughout the organ as greyish foci visible to the naked eye – Malpighian corpuscles. Microscopically these corpuscles contain a central arteriole and in the resting state loose aggregations of lymphoid cells and macrophages. In an immunological reaction the peripheral regions of the corpuscle develop germinal centres while the area around the central arteriole corresponds to the paracortex of the lymph node.

Diffuse lymphoid tissue. In addition to these distinct lymphoid organs there are many aggregations of lymphoid tissue throughout the body, some of which are large and of

41

regular occurrence. The majority of these are associated with the gut and include the *Peyer's patches* – focal aggregations of lymphoid cells beneath the serosa of the small intestine.

Diffuse gut associated lymphoid tissue: diffuse collections of lymphocytes beneath the lamina propria of the small intestine, the tonsils and the vermiform appendix. There are also collections of lymphoid cells in relation to the major air channels of the lung and in conjunction with many of the salivary glands. In addition to these more or less discrete locations for lymphocytes it must be emphasized that lymphoid cells are to be found as constant visitors throughout all the tissues of the body at any one time. The total number of lymphoid cells so located is not precisely known but a not unreasonable guess would be that between 10 and 25% of the total lymphoid mass is diffusely distributed through the tissues at any one time. It is very evident that the cells of the lymphoid system pervade the entire body.

Lymphatic circulation. The distribution and transport of lymphoid cells is accomplished through two major systems: the blood stream and the lymph stream. The blood stream has of course both afferent arterial and efferent venous arms. The lymph stream with respect to the tissues is, however, wholly an efferent drainage channel. The lymph drains the tissues and organs of the body, percolates through lymph nodes and ultimately discharges into major central channels (the thoracic duct is the best known of these and the largest, which in turn empties via the jugular vein into the venous system).

Lymphocytes. The principal cells in immunological reactions are lymphocytes. The classification of lymphocytes used to be rather dull because lymphocytes, like English people to Chinamen, tend to look all alike. Some were larger than others but the typical lymphocyte was a smallish cell (slightly larger than an erythrocyte) composed chiefly of a homogeneous-looking nucleus ensheathed in a sparse rim of cytoplasm containing little in the way of cytoplasmic reticulum and no distinctive organelles. More recently the classification of lymphocytes has become a taxonomist's paradise as their functional heterogeneity is becoming known. The stratification and classification of lymphoid cells has been most closely studied in mice. However, preliminary evidence from a wide variety of other species including man suggests a parallel development. The following description will be based largely upon what is known of the lymphoid system of mice with the understanding that some qualifications may be necessary before application to other species. The major subdivision of lymphoid cells is between those which are primarily responsible for the cell mediated immunities (CMI) and those which are primarily responsible for the humoral immunities. For reasons which will become apparent later, they are often referred to as 'T' and 'B' cells respectively. Further subdivisions can be readily made. For example, subpopulations of B cells may be distinguished by the class of antibody they produce, i.e. IgM, IgG, etc. (Chapter 1), the allotype of antibody and ultimately by the idiotype itself. Moreover, a distinction may be made between cells in the antigen sensitive stage and those differentiating along the pathway that leads to the plasma cell.

Similarly the T cell family includes the recirculating T cell: T cells in the periphery perform a variety of functions, some of which they acquire after exposure to antigen. These functions include cytoxicity, 'helping' antibody formation, graft-versus-host activity (pp. 67 and 79) and in addition probably the regulation of the amplitude of immune reaction (the newly discovered 'regulatory' function of T cells).

Differentiation in the thymus. Both T and B cells appear to arise from a primitive stem cell in the bone marrow, but their pathways of differentiation at once diverge. Bone marrow stem cells of the T line of descent migrate to the thymus where, under the influence of the microenvironment, perhaps abetted by a thymic hormone 'thymosin', they become immature thymocytes. Their cell surfaces change and they acquire characteristic antigens such as theta and LY 1 and in some strains of mice the antigen TL as well. There is at the same time a corresponding reduction in the expression of major histocompatibility antigens (see Chapter 3). Changes of cortisone resistance also accompany the maturation of thymocytes in the thymus; thus administration of cortisone leaves a more mature population in the thymic medulla. Maturation from mature thymocyte to mature recirculating T cell is accompanied by an increase in the resistance to corticosteroid hormones.

Differentiation in the periphery. Following a certain level of maturation within the thymus, T cells, as they are now called (T cell = thymus-derived cell) migrate from the thymus into the periphery. In the first instance they go predominantly to the spleen where they express the cell surface markers LY 1,2,3, and theta, and within the spleen they undergo further maturation. As a result, various subpopulations of T cells are produced, differing in their functional capacity, cell surface markers and homing characteristics. Amongst the subpopulations produced are: (a) the precursors of cytotoxic cells capable of developing into the 'killer cells' of classic cell mediated immunity, directed against certain transplantation antigens (alloantigens). These pre-cytotoxic cells have characteristic cell surface markers, LY 2 and 3, in addition to the theta antigen shared by all peripheral T cells. Pre-cytotoxic cells are amongst the recirculating population of T cells, and have a tendency to home to lymph nodes, rather than to the spleen. (b) The cells active in mixed lymphocyte reactions and graft-versus-host reactions: these are now known to be in a category different from (a) above, since they have a different cell surface marker, namely LY 1. They are the cells which respond by proliferation to certain transplantation antigens, and, in so doing, amplify, or help, the development of the pre-cytotoxic cells, (a) above, into killer cells. (c) The T cells which 'help' in certain B-cell (antibody producing) responses. They also bear the LY 1 surface marker, and it is not yet clear whether they are a separate subpopulation from (b) above. The functionally distinct groups of peripheral T cells, (a) (b) and (c) above, all recirculate throughout the body, including the lymph nodes, in which they comprise the largest proportion of cells. Class (a), the pre-cytotoxic cells, seem to be long-lived and do not require to be constantly replenished from the immature splenic LY 1,2,3 bearing pool. In contrast classes (b) and (c) are relatively short-lived, and they require lifelong replenishment from the splenic LY 1,2,3 bearing pool, which in turn is fed by migration from the thymus. If a mouse, during adult life, has either thymus or spleen removed, T 'helper' function, exemplified by (b) and (c) above, is preferentially impaired. Another functional class of T lymphocytes, that of suppressor or regulator cells, is known to occur and to have great importance in regulating many types of immune function, both humoral and cell mediated. At this time it is not clear whether these suppressor cells belong to a particular subclass, with characteristic cell surface markers, or whether suppressor function is to be found within the subclasses already defined. In some systems there is evidence that suggests that the splenic LY 2,3 bearing pool has suppressor function, whilst in others, it may be that regulation both down (= suppression or antergy) or up (= amplification or synergy) is a function of LY 1,2,3 bearing cells.

B cells. Bone marrow stem cells which take up residence in the *Bursa of Fabricius* (or its mammalian equivalent*) differentiate in to mature B cells which are small lymphocytes whose cell surfaces are theta negative but carry the distinctive marker immunoglobulin. These cells home selectively to the spleen and take up residence. They are also to be found in smaller proportions in other peripheral lymphoid tissues. By contrast to their recirculating T cell counterparts they are relatively sedentary and although they move from one site to another, they do not recirculate in the same way. Inasmuch as the end product of B cell differentiation is the formation of humoral antibody which can act at a considerable

* Although many candidates have been put forward for this office none thus far has been fully acceptable. The term 'B' cell is agreeably ambiguous for it may denote 'bursa-derived', 'bursa-dependent' or 'bone marrow-derived' cells, according to context.

distance from its cell of origin an analogy may be drawn between infantry and artillery. In an immunological assault upon an unwelcome invader (traitorous cells included) T cells are like the infantry. They must move out into the territory combing and searching out the intruder and upon entering an engagement must both give the general alarm and battle at close quarters. B cells are like the artillery. They can safely sit within the fortresses of central lymphoid tissue sending out their destructive missiles which home on their target by means of the critical sensing device of their antibody combining site, and so achieve their destruction at a distance.

Antigen recognition. The way in which B lymphoid cells recognize their antigenic targets seems relatively straightforward because their surfaces are equipped with the exquisitely sensitive and specific antigen-combining sites which antibodies provide. It would be simple if the same mechanism were to operate on behalf of T cells, and indeed immunoglobulin of the IgM class has been identified on the surface membranes of T cells by some workers. However, other workers have failed to confirm these observations and plausible though not necessarily correct alternative explanations for the positive findings have been put forward. Whatever the solution may be it is clear that T cells possess a mechanism of antigen recognition which, if not identical with the antibody combining site, at least shares its exquisite sensitivity and powers of discrimination.

Interaction with antigen. Interaction with antigen in immunogenic form gives rise to a similar sequence of events in cells of both types, i.e. proliferation and further differentiation. Proliferation expands the potentially reactive clone while differentiation is necessary for the evolution of the appropriate effector cell. With B cells the effector cell is a 'plasma cell' which differs from its precursor in having lost surface immunoglobulin, though it possesses a greatly expanded cytoplasm full of endoplasmic reticulum actively synthesizing antibody. Plasma cells are therefore a factory for antibody production and are a relatively short-lived end cell. Occasionally a malignancy, a 'myeloma', arises in plasma cells and when functional can be recognized by the abnormal abundance of immunoglobulin of monoclonal origin in the serum. Tumours of this kind can be experimentally induced and have been extremely useful for the biochemical study of antibody production. Not nearly so much is known about the many kinds of effector cell of T cell origin. However, the large blast-like cell with a high degree of amoeboid mobility can certainly perform one such function: cytotoxicity, i.e. can kill directly (without the collusion of complement). This destruction has been attributed to the release of 'lymphokines' which are highly toxic at close quarters (though some doubt has been thrown on this interpretation), or possibly by some direct mechanical action of the cells themselves. In any event close approximation between activated T cell and target is required.

Interactions between lymphoid cells. In addition to their activities considered severally, it has become increasingly clear that many immunologic functions depend upon the close interaction and co-operation between specialized subpopulations of lymphoid cells.

Lymphoid cells or their products can interact both positively ('synergy') or negatively ('antergy').

Synergy. Synergistic interactions may be either homonomous or heteronomous. In *B-B synergy* for example B cells may interact with other B cells in complement-dependent cell lysis mediated through antibodies, or antibodies produced by different cells and directed towards different cell surface antigens may synergize in the destruction of the cell, e.g. sublytic concentrations of either specificity may produce lysis when combined. *T-T synergy* is a newly described and poorly understood phenomenon. It is clear however that under some circumstances the combination of cells of the mature recirculating type with regulatory cells may produce an effect greater than the sum of their actions individually, e.g. in the graft-versus-host response (Chapter 3). At least two interpretations of this observation are possible. The first rests upon the recruitment of immature and incompetent T cells. The second explanation envisages a regulation of the action of mature recirculating T cells in which the regulating cells themselves take no direct action. At present the latter explanation appears the more likely.

T-B synergy. The discovery that T and B cells could also interact synergistically came as a surprise and discomfiture to some immunologists, for it upset the neat symmetry proposed by those who had thought of a complete distinction between cell mediated and humoral immunities. As often happens in scientific discovery, the crucial observations were made almost simultaneously by a number of investigators working independently in different countries. A relatively small group of antigens characterized by regular and frequent repetitions of the same haptenic configuration can trigger B cells to antibody-production *without* the interposition of T cells. However, the great majority of protein antigens require T cell participation for a complete antibody response. Therefore antigen recognition *per se* is not sufficient: a second signal is necessary to set in train the sequence of B cell differentiation. Some molecules possess intrinsically this ability to trigger B cells: these are the *thymus-independent antigens.* However, the remainder require the help of T cells and are therefore described as *thymus-dependent.* A part of the molecule other than the hapten to which antibody will ultimately be made is often or perhaps invariably the stimulus for T cell participation. The functional role of this other molecular contribution was understood before elucidation of its mechanism and the element responsible for triggering T cells was referred to as the carrier or *schlepper* portion of the molecule. The story of T/B interaction provides a beautiful example of how a sophisticated response requires the co-operation of highly specialized units and may be read as a parable by members of our super-specialized societies.

Antergy. The classical example of *B-B interaction in antergy* is the regulation of antibody production mediated through antibody itself – negative feedback. An attractive explanation of this phenomenon is the competition between preformed antibody and receptors on the B cell surface for antigen; the continued presence of antigen being required for a continued immunological response. In this competition the combining sites which are best adapted, i.e. are most highly specific, will form the most avid bonds with antibody and therefore be at a selective advantage. *B-T antergy* is more commonly known as 'enhancement' (see also Chapter 3).

T-B antergy is a newly described phenomenon in which T cells believed to belong to the regulator subcategory can inhibit or suppress the response of B cells to antigen.

With thymus-dependent antigens this net effect probably occurs through the action of regulatory T cells on helper T cells or directly on B cells themselves. However, as this phenomenon appears also to occur with thymus-independent antigens the direct effect of regulatory T cells on B cells themselves is also possible.

T-T antergy. Suppression of T cell responses during the graft-versus-host reactions and in MLC has been shown to occur as a result of the regulatory action of T cells and there is now some discussion of its playing a part in immunological tolerance (Chapter 3).

Lymphocyte kinetics. In considering the population dynamics of lymphocytes and more especially those of the recirculating T cell we must marvel at the cleverness of the arrangement and can return profitably to the army analogy. In a very real sense continued life or at least health depends upon the outcome of numerous small but continuous engagements against potential invaders at all portals of entry as well as surveyance against treachery from within. In the teleology of the immunological defences the recirculating lymphocyte, a phylogenetically old development, represents an active first line of defence in contrast to the defence in depth and necessarily supportive function of the B cell system. Their continuous percolation through the tissues equips recirculating T cells admirably for their postulated role of surveyance against the development of aberrant (e.g. malignant) cells, and equips them also for a function attributed to them much earlier: a trephocytic function which might also be accompanied by the destruction of senescent cells.

Alterations in kinetics after immunization. In the immune animal the various lymphoid compartments are in kinetic equilibrium but after intentional immunization the dynamics of lymphocytes change in ways important to the development of the subsequent immune response. Prominent amongst these changes is the development of *trapping.* This term refers to the capture or arrest of lymphocytes within lymphoid organs that have been activated by exposure to antigen.

The sequestration of cells from the circulation into the antigen-stimulated lymphoid organ occurs within minutes of antigen's reaching it and operationally may be likened to a closure of outflow while inflow continues. Depending upon such variables as the nature and dose of antigen and the route of administration, trapping lasts for 24 to 48 hours. The functional significance of this kinetic event is that it makes possible the concentration of cells potentially reactive to a particular antigen and therefore an acceleration and augmentation of the immune response. When the trap opens cells temporarily detained but indifferent to the particular antigen are released.

Adjuvants, a heterogeneous group of substances which enhance immune responsiveness, have been shown to be particularly potent in springing the lymphocyte trap. They may act in this way on behalf of antigens which are non-immunogenic through a lack of ability to spring the lymphocyte trap on their own, and in this way confer immunogenicity on otherwise non-immunogenic antigens. A failure of this trapping mechanism would be expected to diminish the effectiveness of the immune response and, indeed, certain advanced tumours in experimental situations can produce this effect, so offering a possible explanation of the immunologically deficient state often observed in animals and man with advanced malignancy. Lymphocyte kinetics is also important in the *propagation of the immune response* for it is clear that an immune reaction initiated in one particular lymph node eventually spreads until the immune state becomes general throughout the body. The sequence of events which accompanies the rejection of an orthotopic skin allograft is particularly instructive (see Chapter 3). After the re-establishment of vascular supply recirculating T lymphocytes enter the graft and the appropriate antigen-sensitive clones affect recognition. Some of these cells travel through the lymphatic channels or draining veins to the regional lymph node where they enter the paracortex and begin the series of maturational steps consisting of division and differentiation. The descendants of these cells enter the efferent lymphatic drainage and are carried to the blood stream where some are widely dispersed throughout the body to other lymphoid organs, while others home selectively to the skin allograft as effector cells and begin the process of graft destruction. This role of the afferent lymphatics and regional nodes was long ago brought to light by the observation that skin allografts enjoyed a prolonged survival when placed on the arm of a woman who had undergone radical mastectomy (including ablation of the lymph nodes on the same side). Moreover, in experimental animals it has been shown very clearly that skin allografts and even xenografts placed within a pedicle are rejected only very slowly through a failure to sensitize, though they are normally susceptible to lymphocytic attack. The curious fact that the genesis of effector T cells requires, or at least proceeds more efficiently, in the microenvironment of lymph nodes was clearly demonstrated by experiments which showed that allograft rejection could be prevented by diverting efferent lymph outside the body. The spread of sensitivity from regional lymphoid organs also occurs in respect of B cell responses. In these responses the relative contributions made by regional immunization and immunization by a 'spillover' of antigen *in situ* cannot be quantified, but here, too, it seems that reactivity is spread around the body by the circulation of B cells. Their descendants may be detected in the blood and lymphatic circulation, and in rats there is some evidence that some B cells may even recirculate like their T counterparts.

An awareness of the dynamic state of the lymphoid system has many *practical implications.* It is becoming increasingly fashionable to study immunological responses *in vitro,* and in the interests of experimental animals well-meaning but misguided souls are attempting to introduce legislation to make the change from *in vivo* to *in vitro* methods, obligatory. From the foregoing discussion, however, it should be clear that an *in vitro* model could not possibly reproduce the kinetic complexities of the situation *in vivo,* and regardless of the ingenuity of design, could tell only part of the story. Moreover, a variety of immunosuppressive manoeuvres depend upon lymphocyte recirculation if they are to work. The most obvious examples are thoracic duct drainage, extra-corporeal irradiation of blood or lymph, and antilymphocyte serum which selectively destroys recirculating lymphocytes.

Other lymphoid cells. The foregoing account of lymphocyte subpopulations has been focussed chiefly on the families of T and B cells. However, there are cells of other types which look like lymphocytes and participate in immune responses, but cannot always be classified as either T or B. Amongst these are 'null' cells which have neither immunoglobulins nor theta on their surfaces, including the lymphocytes which may kill target cells passively coated with antibody through a receptor for the Fc portion of the molecule. To these must at present be added some lymphoid cells found in peritoneal exudate and cerebrospinal fluid. These various cells types are incompletely classified, and the classes to which they belong may well overlap. It is clear, however, that we are just beginning to understand the heterogeneity among lymphoid cells and that until we are very much better informed we shall not fully understand immunological responses.

Macrophages. If the lymphocyte plays the principal part in immunological responsiveness, then the macrophage must certainly receive an award as the best supporting player. If we are incompletely informed about lymphocytes, then we are abysmally ignorant about macrophages. It has been complacently taught that one cell, the macrophage, takes different forms according to its location; there is accordingly a wide variety of synonyms for the same cell: peritoneal macrophage, alveolar macrophage, Kupffer cell in the liver, fixed tissue histiocyte, monocyte in the blood, dendritic macrophage in the lymph node germinal centre, reticular cell, reticulo-endothelial cell, etc. We are led to believe that this protean macrophage can assume very many different forms to achieve a function while preserving its essence.

As with lymphocytes, we are now becoming aware of the *heterogeneity* of macrophages and of the existence of macrophage subpopulations. Macrophages have of course a role independent of the immune response in scavenging debris or damaged cell products. They participate in both the afferent and the efferent (effector) arms of the immunological response. During immunization macrophages capture antigen. In unsensitized animals they can recognize and clear particulate high molecular weight antigens directly. In sensitized animals macrophages passively armed with the appropriate cytophilic antibody are much more efficient and moreover they can then capture antigen of any kind. After digestion further events follow: firstly, macrophages release a factor which springs the lymphocyte trap and secondly, antigen is digested and processed (a process believed by some to entail coupling to RNA) before presentation to the surfaces of T and B cells. This processing-presentation step is an absolute requirement for some antigens and therefore the two-cell model in humoral antibody-production (T-B) must be modified to include the macrophage. Some antigens on the other hand do not require macrophage processing in order to be immunogenic, and processing may, indeed, be detrimental to the immune response. Macrophage participation during the sensitization of T cells is a much less definite affair. However, macrophages appear to be required for the sequence of events which culminate in mixed lymphocyte reactions (see pp. 81, 82) – a T cell-dependent process.

Macrophages also act during the *effector phase* and share with polymorphs the role of destroying antibody-coated bacteria or other single cells, clearing antigen-antibody complexes by phagocytosis and participating in the direct destruction of tumour or allograft target cells, perhaps after being armed by cytophilic antibody of B or perhaps of T cell origin. There is, in addition, a large element of non-specificity in macrophage effector function, for macrophages activated by one form of immunization may perform more effectively upon confrontation by a new type of challenge. The immunopotentiating potency of such agents as *C. parvum* or *M. tuberculosis* vaccines in activating macrophages in this non-specific way may be responsible for their therapeutic efficacy.

Non-specificity of inflammation. Whereas the exquisite specificity of the immune response has been repeatedly emphasized, it is nevertheless true that the inflammatory element of the final effector phase common to a wide variety of immunological reactions is largely non-specific. The action of pharmacologically active lymphokines, lysomal enzymes released by polymorphs, activation of the complement sequence, and the non-specific activation of macrophages all enter into inflammation and may damage cells in their neighbourhood. This potential for host tissue damage during immune responses may have considerable relevance to autoimmunity (p. 132).

E.M.L.
E.S

CHAPTER THREE
Transplantation Immunity, Immunosuppression and Tolerance

Transplantation immunity is the form of CMI (see p. 7) which normally prohibits the transplantation of living tissues between two different human beings, chickens, goldfish or mice. This prohibition applies to any two members of ordinary outbred populations of all vertebrate animals (including fish and even cyclostomes) which have been studied in sufficient detail to make a judgement possible. Grafts between two individuals belonging to the same species are now referred to as 'allografts' (formerly as 'homografts'). Grafts between members of different species are 'xenografts' (formerly 'heterografts'). Grafts transplanted from one part to another of a single individual are referred to as 'autografts'. When donor and recipient are identical twins or are as closely alike genetically as inbreeding can make them (see below) the grafts are referred to as 'syngeneic'. Although common

in the older literature, the adjectives 'heterologous', 'homologous' and 'isologous' are now
seldom used for the relationships described as
xenogeneic, allogeneic and syngeneic respectively; nevertheless 'homologous' is still widely
used to refer to the relation between an
antibody and the antigen to which it corresponds.

Although not yet in clinical use the allograft
of skin is that which has been most widely
used for experimental purposes. The natural
history of a skin allograft on an animal which
has not previously received grafts from a
related donor source is much the same
throughout vertebrate animals: the graft is
vascularized within a few days by the process
of *abbouchement,* i.e. the end to end anasto-
mosis of vessels in the graft bed with vessels
already present in the graft. Within six or
seven days the graft vessels become grossly
engorged and dilated, lymphocytes pass
through the vessel walls and penetrate all
parts of the graft, lymphatics become
prominent and are seen to be crowded with
lymphocytes. The inner layers of the epidermal epithelium begin to lose their attachment
to the underlying corium and start to break
up. Meanwhile the blood circulation comes
slowly to a standstill and the graft dies. In the
next stage epidermal epithelium from the
surrounding skin of the recipient cuts into and
undermines the dying graft which is eventually
sloughed off as a dried scab. The process of

undermining may occur at such a level of the graft that the host's epithelium covers much of the remaining part of graft collagen, so giving a fairly plausible imitation of a graft that is still alive – the commonest cause of a mistaken belief in an allograft's continued survival. When donor and recipient differ from each other at 'strong' histocompatibility loci (see below) the process of rejection is normally complete by 11–12 days after grafting or even sooner.

If such a skin allograft is transplanted to an animal already sensitized by a prior exposure to tissues from the same donor source, its natural history is somewhat different: vascularization is imperfect and lymphocytic infiltration much reduced. The circulation comes much more rapidly to a standstill and the graft suffers an ischaemic death. This is the rather oddly-named 'second set' reaction, so called because it was first studied in detail in organisms large enough to receive a first population followed by a second population of small separate skin allografts ('pinch' grafts). In a highly sensitive individual the vascularization of a second graft is so imperfect that it can be regarded as virtually avascular and can hardly be said to survive at all except as a sort of tissue culture *in vivo*. This is the so-called 'white graft' reaction, which is not qualitatively different from the ordinary second set reaction, though it is markedly more intense. There has been some controversy about whether the second set reaction is something equivalent to the humoral secondary response (see paragraph 3 on p. 15), i.e. represents a reawakening of the host response, or whether it is merely a passive indicator, as a skin test might be, of a pre-existing state of sensitivity. Whatever may be the truth with regard to the CMI element of the response, there is no doubt that there is a true secondary response in the formation of humoral antibodies, for allografts produce not only a CMI but also an antibody response of exactly the same specificity.

By contrast to passive humoral immunity (see p. 26) sensitivity to allografts cannot be conferred upon a secondary host by serum transfusions from an actively immunized serum donor. On the contrary, the effect of these humoral antibodies is, if anything, to impede the CMI element of the response – the phenomenon of 'enhancement' (see pp. 100 and 108). Sensitivity can be conferred upon a secondary host only by a transference of lymphoid cells from lymph nodes or spleen or by a transfusion of blood lymphocytes. Immunity acquired in this way is said to be 'adoptive' in origin, to distinguish it from conventional passive immunity and from active immunity. Adoptive immunity lasts as long as active immunity. It sometimes takes better effect when the recipient is lightly irradiated as if to make room for the newly introduced cells. When a second allograft of the right specificity is put upon an animal which is thereupon adoptively immunized, it is tempting to believe that the transferred leucocytes themselves congregate around and destroy the graft, but it seems more likely that the transferred cells travel first to lymph nodes where they divide to give rise to progeny that home on the graft.

Transplantation antigens. Some of the antigens associated one way or another with transplantation reactions are related not merely functionally but also genetically. These are the 'strong' transplantation antigens. They illustrate a principle first enunciated by R. A. Fisher in tending to congregate along a single stretch of chromosome which carries the genetic determinants of the major histocompatibility complex (MHC) in all the animals in which it has been sought. Priority of analysis, as usual on these occasions, belongs to the mouse, but no final pronouncement on the detailed structure of this stretch of chromosome can yet be made. The subject owes its complexity to the fact that there are many different modalities of allogeneic reactivity of which straightforward graft rejection, as typified by the rejection of skin allografts, is only one. Among the others mentioned above are: the formation of humoral antibodies that accompanies graft rejection; graft-versus-host reactivity in all its many manifestations (pp. 79-80) and the stimulation of lymphoid cells to divide in the mixed leucocyte reaction

(MLR). In each such reaction we may identify the antigen either as the agent that excites an immune response or as the target of that response.

The 'classical' antigens which play so large a part in governing the outcome of tumour and tissue transplantations in mice were worked out partly by the most laborious genetical tests with transplanted tumours and partly by the agglutination of red cells (which was, in fact, the means by which the principal histocompatibility genes of mice were first discovered, by Peter Gorer). These antigens form a family united by the property that they can be serologically defined and are accordingly called SD antigens. Some other antigens are identified by the performance of lymphocytes in one allogeneic confrontation or another: MLR for example, or GVH reactivity. These are the 'lymphocyte' defined or LD antigens.

In mice and some other animals the genes governing the inheritance of SD differences are clustered at the two ends of the stretch of chromosome referred to above – in mice the K and D ends. Between these two ends in mice are the genes governing MLR and also the reactivity towards a variety of synthetic antigens. These latter are the *Ir* genes. In man and in some other animals the Ir genes and LD antigen determinants lie *outside* the chromosome stretch bounded by SD determinants although they are closely linked. In addition to these, SD genes coding for transplantation antigens are also found on chromosomes other than that occupied by a major histocompatibility complex, and these are sometimes referred to as 'minor histocompatibility genes', but their effects are additive and a sum of disparities at minor loci may have the effect of a major histocompatibility difference.

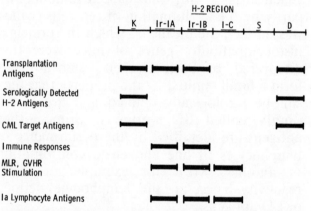

Fig. 4. Diagram illustrating the H-2 region of the ninth linkage group in the mouse: illustrating the relative positions occupied by the K, D and I regions. For description, see text.

Our present conception of the interrelations of LD and SD genetic determinants is shown in Fig. 4.

As things stand at present there is no certainty about what form of matching should best be used to prolong the life of allografts to the utmost; indeed, the development of more and more powerful immunosuppressive procedures has made some surgeons retreat into the sceptical position of saying that no matching of any kind is really necessary. It would indeed not be necessary if conventional immunosuppression were as powerful as that which can be secured by antilymphocyte globulin (p. 99) and could be long sustained, for ALG makes possible the transplantation even of xenografts. Another category of antigens which has become increasingly prominent in transplantation work is the *tissue specific* antigen which differs from one individual to another. There is no reason why such antigens should not act in the rejection of allografts, and some of them – among them a skin specific antigen – are known to do so. The term 'differentiation antigen' applies generally to all antigens which distinguish one tissue or cell lineage from another or one subclass of tissue from another – e.g. one lymphocyte class from another. Differentiation antigens are of special importance in experimental work and they often serve as markers of cells that could not otherwise be identified: a consideration which applies with special force to cells of the lymphoid family.

Identification of the alloantigens that may play a part in determining the outcome of transplantations is one of the most rapidly growing areas of modern transplantation biology.

Chemical nature of transplantation antigens. A subject on which no final pronouncement can be made is the chemical nature of the various categories of antigens involved in alloimmune reactivity. Of these, most important from a practical point of view are those which arouse transplantation immunity and which, appropriately used, may produce transplantation tolerance. Most methods of testing for antigenicity – e.g. the injection into mice of putatively antigenic matter to see if grafts transplanted on later occasions are rejected in the accelerated or 'second set' style – are quantitatively insensitive and marred by poor dose/response relationships. More, perhaps, is to be expected from the study of specific inhibition of agglutination or cytotoxicity reactions or from the use of those hypersensitivity reactions akin to the tuberculin reaction which good performers in reactions of this kind, such as guinea pigs, may be made to display.

The immunization process. It was at one time taken for granted that antigens issued from the graft into the regional lymphatics and thus found their way into the regional nodes, which underwent the changes characteristic of antigenic activation, and it is certainly true that in areas devoid of or deprived of lymphatics the allograft reaction is greatly impaired. It is now coming quite widely to be thought that the antigenicity of the graft is in large part to be attributed to the leucocytes ('passenger leucocytes') that are inevitably carried over with it, and some of the antigenic characteristics of the graft can indeed be made to vary with the genetic provenance of the bone marrow of the animal from which the grafts were removed. An alternative view, widely referred to in the literature and still under analysis, goes under the name of *peripheral sensitization*: in this view the cells that initiate the allograft reaction by recognizing antigen and taking the first steps in reacting against it are circulating peripheral blood lymphocytes; these are immunologically activated by contact with the graft endothelium or other graft elements, whereupon they find their way into the lymphatics and so into the regional nodes. In experiments in which skin allografts or xenografts in guinea pigs are transplanted to flaps of skin deprived of lymphatic drainage, breakdown is greatly delayed in onset and survival is very much prolonged. Breakdown eventually occurs nevertheless, and this must almost certainly be the consequence of peripheral immunization.

Breakdown process. Although it is well known that breakdown is accompanied by a local congregation of lymphocytes, the mechanism by which allografts are destroyed is still not understood. However, lymphocytes from sensitized individuals can be made to attack and destroy target cells *in vitro* in complement-free media and if this is a faithful representation of what occurs *in vivo* then it can be said with confidence that the process is not complement-dependent, but even in the *in*

71

vivo context the exact nature of the engagement between the sensitized lymphocyte and its target is not known. It cannot, however, be long before the refinement of *in vitro* methods makes it clear.

The 'self + x' hypothesis. One person's organs must have much the same chemical make-up as another's. What makes A's skin antigenic to B must therefore be the presence of something extra in A – something lacking in B. An authority on CMI has proposed that all CMI is aroused by antigens of the 'self + x' category, and this hypothesis applies with special force to the haptenic chemicals such as dinitrochlorobenzene and o-cresol which sensitize only after attachment to the recipient's protein – a palpable 'self + x' situation.

Organ specific alloantigens. It was at one time believed that all nucleated tissue cells in the body have the same make-up of alloantigens, but it is now realized that organ-specific antigens may differ from one individual to another and may thus act as transplantation antigens. Skin possesses one such 'differentiation antigen' and lymphoid tissues several others (see Chapter 2).

Genetics and the allograft reaction. When the members of a laboratory population of, for example, guinea pigs, rats or mice are inbred by successive sibling or parent/offspring matings for upwards of fifty generations, the members of the population come to resemble each other – differences of sex apart – almost as closely as if they were identical twins. In setting up or maintaining such an inbred strain it is most important that the parents of each successive generation should be chosen *at random*, for if the first female to become pregnant is chosen to be the parent of the next generation it is inevitable that there should be some selection for heterozygosity, and the purpose of inbreeding will be defeated. Grafts exchanged between members of strictly inbred populations are 'syngeneic' and will behave essentially like autografts. Grafts between identical twins are also, of course, syngeneic and their success is limited by surgical and physiological considerations only. The relationship between identical twins may be said to define one end of a wide spectrum of affinities of which the other end is occupied by xenografts, e.g. grafts from mouse to rabbit or from chimpanzee to man. In summary, xeno-grafts may be said to excite the same kind of reaction as allografts, only more so. With xenografts, however, there is no doubt at all that humoral antibodies are important effec-tors of the immune response. There is, never-theless, an important CMI component in the reaction against xenografts, because their survival may be prolonged by immunosup-pressive agents (see below) that act selectively upon CMI.

There is one important exception to the general principle that grafts are freely inter-changeable between members of highly inbred strains: in some strains of mice females regularly reject grafts transplanted from males of the same inbred strain, after periods ranging from 15 to 50 days. Expression of the male-specific antigens is programmed by a gene on the Y chromosome characteristic of males.

Genetic 'laws' of transplantation. The generalizations which now follow were established by early workers on the transplantation of tumours, particularly at Bar Harbor, Maine, though most of the 'laws' they established are known to hold good of the transplantation of normal tissues, including skin. With the exception noted above, grafts can be exchanged freely between members of a highly inbred strain and between monozygotic twins. They may also be transplanted from members of either parental strain to the hybrid first generation (F_1) progeny of a cross between two such inbred strains. Indeed, F_1 hybrids are universal recipients in the microcosm of mice comprising two parental inbred strains, their F_1 progeny, all possible backcross progeny and the F_2 or later generations derived from mating together the F_1 and so on repeatedly. On the other hand, grafts from parental strains take and survive in only a limited proportion of F_2 and backcross progeny, and the ratio of takes to failures makes it possible to determine the number of Mendelian factors involved in allograft rejection in any two inbred strains. The traditional factorial explanation of these

74

results runs as follows: the antigenicity of the graft is determined by one or more members of a complex of dominant genes which if present in the donor of the graft and absent from its recipient will cause breakdown. The F_1 progeny of a cross between homozygous mice are universal recipients because they contain representatives of all the genes and therefore all the antigens present in either of their parents. If, however, the parental strains differ at a number of loci then segregation will occur in the mating together of F_1 hybrids to form an F_2 progeny. If, for example, the parental strains differ by one 'histocompatibility' gene then in the F_2 generation the ratio of takes to non-takes will be 3:1. As the following example makes clear, all this follows from elementary Mendelian rules. With this purely formal example we may neglect all gene pairs in respect of which the two parental strains are identical, for these will be identical in the F_1 and the F_2 generations. Suppose that a parental strain I has the following make-up of histocompatibility genes: A A B B c c, and that a second strain II has the make-up: A A B B C C, then the F_1 progeny $I \times II$ will all have the make-up: A A B B C c. When these F_2 progeny are mated together the following classes of offspring will be produced.

A A B B C C	1/4 lack the gene C.
A A B B C c	1/4 lack the gene c. 2/4 are
A A B B C c	hybrids like their parents
A A B B c c	and possess both C and c.

Suppose now that both C and c each determine the formation of an antigen singly sufficient to cause the breakdown of an allograft on a recipient in which those genes are absent. If this is so, it will be clear that grafts transplanted from strain I or strain II upon the F_2 generation will fail only in that one quarter of the progeny in which genes c or C respectively are lacking – a typical 3:1 Mendelian ratio of successes to failures.

Number of histocompatibility loci: strong and weak antigens. Analysis of the number of loci in mice involved in skin or tumour transplantation immunity by the type of segregation analysis illustrated above originally gave figures of twenty upwards. Subsequently genetic methods of isolating histocompatibility (H) loci have identified a minimum of thirty-five. The antigens they code for are divided into two classes: strong, as exemplified by the MHC (H-2 in the mouse, HLA in man) – see also pp. 66–8 and Fig. 4 – and weak or minor transplantation antigens (p. 67). In the MHC, the strong antigens are coded by loci which tend to congregate at the K and D ends of the complex (Fig. 4). The loci coding for weak antigens are on a number of other chromosomes and are less complex in their arrangement than the MHC. Strong (i.e. H-2) transplantation antigens bring about the breakdown of skin grafts in about ten days whilst weak (i.e. non H-2) transplantation antigens, singly at least, may provoke a very prolonged rejection, taking several weeks. However, the effect of a number of weak antigens together is cumulative, and when skin is grafted between two H-2 identical strains such as C3H and CBA, which differ at a number of minor H loci, the rejection time is not much longer than that for strong, H-2 antigens.

Histocompatibility antigens and polymorphism. The fact that there is no convincing evidence of the take of a skin allograft transplanted between members of an ordinary outbred population shows that polymorphism with respect to the antigens that determine the outcome of transplantation reactions · is very fine-grained. The selective forces which maintain this polymorphism are not yet known; nor is the survival-value or 'purpose' of transplantation immunity yet understood except in so far as it may be a by-product of immunological surveyance (see pp. 105, 133).

Other Manifestations of Allogeneic Reactivity

The rejection of allografts is not the only manifestation of transplantation immunity and the next few paragraphs deal with other manifestations of the same type of incompatibility, viz.: delayed-type hypersensitivity reactions and graft-versus-host (GVH) reactions including the normal lymphocyte transfer reaction. Finally, mention will be made of mixed leucocyte reactions (MLR).

Allograft reactions and delayed-type reac-

tivity. It is a matter of some theoretical interest that in animals such as human beings and guinea pigs which are specially liable to the cutaneous inflammation that accompanies delayed-type hypersensitivity reactions (see paragraph 2 on p. 10) an allograft reaction can be made to manifest itself as a delayed-type hypersensitivity. Suppose that a guinea pig R has been sensitized by the grafting of tissues from a donor guinea pig D. Delayed cutaneous inflammatory reactions of two kinds may now be made to manifest themselves:

1. A *direct* hypersensitivity reaction when antigenic matter from D, whether in the form of a cellular extract or of living cells, is injected intracutaneously into R.
2. A *transfer reaction* when regional lymph node cells or peritoneal or blood lymphocytes from R are injected into the skin of D.

Both reactions have the tempo and general character of delayed-type hypersensitivity reactions, but the transfer reaction is very difficult to interpret because the transfer of lymphoid cells from R into D is accompanied by a congregation of D cells around the point of injection. Direct reactions excited by cellular extracts are much easier to interpret and have been put to good use in tumour immunology (see Chapter 4) and in the characterization of transplantation antigens.

Graft-versus-host (GVH) reactions. When a graft contains or consists of lymphoid cells, lymphocytes or in general of immunologically competent cells, it should in theory be able to counterattack the tissues of its host by a sort of allograft reaction-in-reverse. This theoretical possibility can be realized only when the host cannot defend itself, i.e. cannot destroy the intruding allogeneic lymphoid cells before they do harm. The characteristic situations that make GVH reactions possible are when lymphoid cells derived from members of parental strains of inbred mice are injected into F_1 hybrids (which, as explained above, cannot reject them) and when lymphoid cells are injected into very young animals or into animals which have been the subject of vigorous immunosuppressive procedures, or other procedures designed to make them tolerant of the donor cells (see pp. 85-6). GVH reactions manifest themselves in quite a variety of different ways:

1. *Runt disease*, a wasting disease brought about by the injection of adult allogeneic lymphoid cells into newborn rats or mice and characterized by severe retardation of growth, many autoimmune manifestations and a general lymphoid hypoplasia.

2. *Splenomegaly*, a gross enlargement of the spleens of young mice or chick embryos that follows the injection into

them of allogeneic lymphoid cells. A variant of the same response is that in which a regional lymph node - e.g. the popliteal lymph node of a mouse or rat enlarges greatly in response to a regional inoculation of allogeneic lymphoid cells.

3. *Secondary radiation sickness* is the debility which gives rise to the puzzling 'late deaths' that occur when mice exposed to lethal doses of whole-body irradiation (e.g. 700–900 r) are rescued by the inoculation of allogeneic bone marrow cells, which inevitably contain lymphocytes. A sickness of the same kind - also often fatal - may also occur when lymphoid cells from inbred parental strain mice are injected into an F_1 hybrid between that strain and any other. As explained above (see paragraph 2 on p. 74), such hybrids are immunologically defenceless against parental strain tissues.

4. *The 'normal lymphocyte transfer' (NLT) reaction* that occurs when normal adult allogeneic lymphocytes are injected into the skins of chickens, hamsters or guinea pigs. The natural history of an NLT reaction in guinea pigs is as follows. A first inflammatory response occurs 24–26 hours after the injection of allogeneic lymphocytes; this remains stationary for a day or two but from the third day onwards flares up to form a much more severe inflammatory lesion,

whereupon the inflammation rather suddenly fades out. This second inflammatory episode is at least partly due to a direct hypersensitivity reaction (see above) on the part of the recipient, and the fade out is certainly due to the recovery of the recipient's immunological competence. An NLT reaction does not show up at all clearly except in recipient guinea pigs which have themselves been subjected to whole-body irradiation (600 r) in order to prevent the prompt rejection of the injected lymphoid cells. The nature of this second inflammatory episode of an NLT reaction will be discussed later under the heading of 'Immunosuppression'.

P.B.M.

5. *Mixed lymphocyte reactions.* When lymphocytes from two unrelated individuals are mixed in culture the cells interact and lymphocyte stimulation occurs: after four to seven days lymphocytes develop into the 'blast' form and divide. Visible signs of this stimulation are enlargement of the cells accompanied by the formation of pyroninophilic and often vacuolated cytoplasm, and the coming of nucleoli into prominence. Active nucleic acid and protein synthesis are followed shortly by cell division. The degree of activation of lymphocytes is almost invariably measured in terms of

the uptake of tritiated thymidine into DNA as determined by scintillation counting. Interaction requires cell/cell contact between actively metabolizing and genetically different lymphocytes, but it is not necessary for the cell donors to have been sensitized beforehand by each other's antigens. The reaction between lymphocytes from different donors appears to depend on genetic disparity in respect of certain antigens of the major histocompatibility complex, so the MLR procedure is potentially useful as an *in vitro* indicator of certain types of allo-incompatibility. As described above, activation is reciprocal - lymphocytes from both donors act as antigens and as responders so both undergo activation. To make the test asymmetrical or one-way, and thus distinguish between reactions of donor and of recipient, lymphocytes from only one of the donors may be irradiated or treated with mito-mycin-C (a toxic antibiotic often used as an immunosuppressive agent). This refinement is obligatory because the information specially sought is whether or not lymphocytes of the recipient will react upon the antigens of a graft donor.

S.K.

Immunological Tolerance*

Immunological tolerance – a state of induced specific immunological non-reactivity – was first brought to prominence by experiments on tissue transplantation; but a phenomenon no longer distinguished from it in principle was first described in 1949 as 'immunological paralysis', a term used to refer to a state of affairs in which mice respond by antibody formation to microgram or even nanogram doses of type-specific pneumococcal poly-saccharides, but respond to milligram doses by entering into a state in which they neither form antibodies on that occasion nor upon later rechallenge. Among other phenomena thought to be cognate with this remarkable elimination of a specific immunological reactivity are:

1. The specific non-reactivity established in mice by the injection into them of purified, clean, aggregate-free solutions of bovine gamma globulin.
2. The state of unresponsiveness brought about in guinea pigs by a systemic injection of chemicals such as orthocresol or dinitrochlorobenzene which would have aroused strong delayed hypersensitivity reactions if they had been applied in the conventional way to the skin.

* The concept of self-tolerance and its relation to the immunological diseases discussed on p.121.

'Paralysis' is now widely used to refer to states of non-reactivity engendered by and enjoyed by well-defined antigens but 'tolerance' remains in general use in the context of transplantation.

Transplantation tolerance. In retrospect the sequence of observations which led to the recognition of the phenomenon of transplantation tolerance can be seen to have a logical connectedness which was far from obvious at the time. Important steps in the formulation of the idea were as follows:

1. The discovery by livestock geneticists in Wisconsin that cattle twins contain mixtures of each other's red blood corpuscles, i.e. a certain proportion – not necessarily a majority – of their 'own' corpuscles mixed with red cells belonging genetically to their partner. Animals containing cells derived from two distinct zygote lineages are referred to as 'chimeras'. It is very relevant that cattle twins had long been known to be synchorial, i.e. to be such that they exchange blood and evidently blood-forming cells too before birth. (All chicken and some sheep twins are synchorial; so also, though very much more rarely, are twin human beings.)

2. Attempts to distinguish monozygotic and dizygotic twins in cattle by the

reciprocal interchange of skin grafts showed that dizygotic twins – even when of different sex – would accept skin grafts from each other instead of rejecting them rather violently as ordinary siblings do.

Experiments in Prague and in University College London were then directed towards trying to reproduce in experimental animals the phenomenon that occurs by a natural accident in twin cattle.

3. In Prague it was shown that if a vascular bridge was established between two embryonated hen's eggs by interposing embryonic tissue between exposed areas of their highly vascular choriollantoic membranes, the chicks after hatching would accept grafts from each other and were incapable of making haemagglutinins against each other's red cells.

4. In University College London it was shown that if a miscellany of cells and tissue fragments from adult A-strain mice were injected into CBA mouse fetuses, then when they grew up mice so inoculated would accept A-strain skin grafts later in life for much longer than would otherwise have been the case.

All these experiments were technically very difficult, but persistence with them was encouraged first of all by the virtually complete certainty that they would succeed if technical difficulties could be overcome and secondly by the attractiveness of Burnet and Fenner's theory of immunity. According to this, the distinction between 'self' and 'non-self' components is crucial, so that a mechanism must exist for annulling any possible reactivity towards 'self' components. Nevertheless, the success of the University College experiments must be regarded in retrospect as something of a fluke: the type of cell used for the fetal inoculum was not in fact at all conducive to the induction of tolerance. It would have been a natural and ostensibly a wiser choice to use *lymphoid* cells from the strain of the future graft donor, but had this been done 'runt disease' or some other variant of graft-versus-host reactions (see pp. 79-80) would have ruined the experiments and the discovery of transplantation tolerance would have been delayed still further. It should however be noted that the experiments carried out in Prague on embryonic parabiosis were not open to this objection because the partners in the parabiosis were not yet immunologically mature.

Characteristics of tolerance. Tolerance is marked by the following properties:

1. Tolerance is induced by antigen. This is one reason why it has been thought expedient to draw a distinction between immunogens on one hand - substances

which excite an immunological response – and antigens in a more general sense which will certainly include their acting in a tolerance-inducing capacity (see p. 83). Substances enjoying this property or acting in this latter capacity have sometimes been referred to as 'tolerogens'. Substances such as bovine gamma globulin (BGG) are not immunogenic in mice, but can be made so by incorporation into adjuvants – notably into Freund's adjuvant which consists of vegetable oil and a wetting agent with or without the addition of dead mycobacteria. As explained above (p. 86), to act as an immunogen a substance must be antigenic and must also enjoy the property of 'adjuvanticity'. Intrinsic adjuvanticity may turn on the ability of an antigenic substance to engage some of the ancillary cells (perhaps macrophages) which play a part in the immunological response or to trap reactive lymphoid cells (p. 54) from the circulation.

2. The state of tolerance is assessed by challenging an organism with the antigen to which it is supposedly non-reactive. Tolerance exists in all degrees, so that the response to this antigenic challenge varies from zero to something little short of normal.

3. The maintenance of the tolerant state

depends upon the continued presence of the antigen that aroused it.

4. Tolerance may be brought to an end and normal reactivity reinstated by adoptive immune cell transfers (p. 27), i.e. by the injection of normal (and necessarily syngeneic) lymphoid cells into the tolerant subject. Another means by which tolerance may sometimes be brought to an end is by active immunization with an antigen overlapping in specificity with that which aroused tolerance.

Age and dosage phenomena. In the induction of transplantation tolerance by the inoculation of very young animals, 'the earlier the better' was thought to be a reliable general rubric. The older literature hints that over a certain age animals become no longer susceptible to the induction of tolerance and that in the course of development they go through a 'neutral period' during which the presentation of antigen arouses neither tolerance nor immunity. Neither of these notions has withstood critical investigation. 'The earlier the better' is difficult to reconcile with the fact that fusion of egg cells or young embryos to form so-called 'tetraparental' mice produces very variable results in terms of transplantation tolerance. Furthermore, in the context of transplantation tolerance the neutral period has no absolute significance: the time at which it ends is a function of the dosage of cells used to induce the tolerance state. However, the age at which it remains feasible to induce tolerance is a function of the rate of maturation of the immunological response system in each species. Guinea pigs and ungulates are born in the relatively mature state and already enjoy a high degree of immunological competence. It is therefore specially difficult to induce transplantation tolerance as late as at birth. Nevertheless, the existence of red-cell chimeras and the mutual tolerance of synchorial human and cattle twins shows that the tolerance principle is no less true of these larger animals than it is of mice. Induction of transplantation tolerance in adult animals depends upon the heroic use of immunosuppressive agents (see below). Research in the radiobiology unit at Harwell showed that mice rescued from otherwise lethal doses of whole-body X or gamma irradiation by an inoculation of allogeneic bone marrow cells would accept skin grafts from mice of the strain of the bone marrow donors. By such means it was even possible to cause mice to accept xenografts. In radiation-induced tolerance, however, the question naturally arises whether the ostensibly tolerant state is in reality simulated by the virtual destruction of all the host's immunologically competent cells and their replacement by cells of the genotype of the graft donor. The same interpretation could apply also, at least in part, to mice in which the blood-forming elements are restored by hybrid allogeneic marrow cells in order to avoid the complications of secondary radiation sickness (see p. 80). Many immunosuppressive procedures other than irradiation can be used to abet the induction of tolerance – especially the use of antilymphocyte serum (see below), but immunosuppressive steroids have not been shown to enjoy this property.

Antigen dosage. The old idea that a high dose of antigen was unconditionally necessary for the induction of tolerance has given way to the discovery that tolerance may be induced in two zones of dosage: the conventional high dose, and a repetition of very low doses – which in the perhaps special case of flagellin from *salmonella adelaide* may be as low as nanogram quantities. However, no one has yet published a successful record of the induction of transplantation tolerance at a low zone of dosage – an important subject for future research.

The mechanism of tolerance (see also pp. 101, 121). It is generally agreed that the induction of tolerance by the injection of allogeneic cells into very young warm-blooded animals is a simulation of the process which, according to Burnet's famous hypothesis, annuls an organism's reaction to self components. Unfortunately this parallel does not take us very far because both processes are equally mysterious. It is universally agreed, however, that no theory of the immunological response will pass muster unless it accounts intercurrently for tolerance as well. Evaluated by this criterion, Burnet's theory of tolerance is still the most satisfactory. Burnet's clonal selection theory of immunity was first devised in order to get round the difficulty made clear by molecular genetics (see p. 5) that antigen cannot inform the structure of an antibody molecule: the amino acid sequence of antibody must therefore be prescribed in nucleic acid. Broadly speaking there are two possibilities, therefore. Either the zygote contains the genetic information necessary to underwrite the formation of antibodies so that this information is present in all the cells – including' lymphocytes – descended from it, with the effect that antigen acts essentially as an embryonic inducer – calling forth one rather than another of the potentialities already enjoyed by the reacting cell; or, alternatively, that the new genetic information is amassed during an animal's lifetime by a mutational process which leads to the formation of a great variety of lymphoid cell clones, each with its own special reaction capability. Mutation may be defined as the coming into being of new genetic information, so to describe the new reaction capabilities as mutational in origin is purely verbal. The second possibility is that which Burnet envisaged in his clonal selection hypothesis: tolerance is the consequence of some special sensitivity of one such clone of cells to antigen, as a consequence of which the entire clone is eliminated and the reaction it would otherwise have empowered is eliminated from the organism's repertoire. If this hypothesis is true it follows that there can be no such thing as a tolerant *cell* – a question that has not yet been decisively answered. If on the other hand all the necessary genetic information is present in the zygote and all its descendants, the inception of tolerance must represent a physiological change in cells that would otherwise have been capable of mounting an immune response. If this is so, then such objects as tolerant cells should exist – so that the question of whether or not tolerant cells exist can again seem to be a crucial one.

There are, however, still more general questions we may ask about the nature of tolerance. From the earliest days of the research into tolerance it was perhaps too readily assumed that the tolerant state represented a total absence of an immunological reactivity – the more or less complete erasure of one specific immunological performance from the organism's repertoire. The reasons for taking this view were (a) the reinstatement of normal reactivity in tolerant mice by the injection of normal syngeneic lymphoid cells and (b) the fact that a variety of the most refined tests for immunological competence failed to reveal any specific immunological capability in the cells of genuinely tolerant mice. A good deal of surprise was aroused, therefore, by the claim that so far from being *essentially* non-reactive, tolerant mice did, in fact, contain hostile lymphoid cells capable of reacting upon antigen, but that these lymphoid cells were prevented from doing so by the interposition of a serum factor – a 'blocking' factor – of unknown nature, possibly an antigen-antibody complex. Recent experiments have not, however, borne out this interpretation, though it is quite possible that blocking factors have a part to play in tolerance under certain circumstances, particularly in the notoriously precarious state of partial tolerance and when an abundance of antigen has access to the general circulation. The most important antithesis in current discussions of the nature of tolerance is between tolerance conceived as essential non-reactivity on the one hand or on the other hand as a state actively maintained by inhibitory factors in serum or perhaps by action of suppressor T cells (see section on T-T antergy in Chapter 2, p. 53).

Immunosuppression and Immunosuppressive Agents

The success of transplantation in clinical practice depends upon the judicious use of immunosuppressive procedures, i.e. of procedures which weaken one or other arm of the immunological response. The pattern of immunosuppressive treatment that has come to be regarded as orthodox in transplantation practice is a combination of Imuran (azathio-prine) with corticosteroids. The uses of immunosuppression are, however, by no means confined to transplantation (see Chapter 5).

Because of the exigent demands of clinical transplantation the goal of most immunosup-pressive procedures has usually been the inhibition of CMI.

The suppression of antibody formation is a somewhat ambiguous ambition because although it may promote CMI by countering 'enhancement', most protective immunity against micro-organisms rests on humoral antibody formation. The suppression of humoral antibody formation would certainly be necessary if xenografts were ever to be used, because antibodies play an important part in their rejection.

Specificity of immunosuppression. The immunosuppressed state in which an organism's response to only one particular antigen is eliminated from its repertoire is known as a state of 'tolerance' or 'paralysis' – the subject of the preceding section. Tolerance is a very special state of affairs because the immuno-suppressive agent is antigen itself, though in adults its use must be abetted by the use of immunosuppressive agents. However, most immunosuppressive agents are not specific, even in the very undemanding sense of acting only upon the immunological response rather than upon any other physiological capabilities.

Irradiation with X-rays or gamma rays is notorious for its inhibitory effect upon proliferative tissues generally, and in particular those of the haematopoietic system.

Modern research upon immunosuppressive agents is, in effect, a search for procedures or agents which are not only restricted in their actions to the immunological response, but affect only one arm of it, e.g. CMI, rather than another. Research on immunosuppression is, nevertheless, still almost wholly empirical and will remain so until someone has propounded a viable theory of the endogenous control of the immune response upon which theoretically well-founded immunosuppressive or immuno-potentiating procedures may be based.

Classes of immunosuppressive agents. Immunosuppressive agents will be considered briefly under the following headings:

1. Ionising radiations.
2. Corticosteroids.
3. Antiproliferative agents.
4. Antilymphocyte serum.
5. Homologous antibody.

1. *Ionising radiations,* particularly X-rays and gamma rays, have a powerful immunosuppressive effect when applied to the whole body in dosages of the order of hundreds of rads. The effect is upon both CMI and humoral immunity, but where, as in transplantation immunity, the two go hand in hand, the effect

is greater upon humoral immunity. The humoral secondary response, and the 'second set' response of animals already exposed to transplantation antigens, are less affected than the corresponding first responses. Ionising radiations are essentially antiproliferative in action, i.e. they do not affect any characteristically immunological performance of the cell.

Thymectomized animals in which haematopoiesis has been gravely impaired by whole-body irradiation can be kept alive only by the inoculation of bone marrow cells – preferably syngeneic to avoid complications of chronic GVH disease (see paragraph 2 on page 80). Experimental animals restored in this way suffer a radical and long-lasting impairment of CMI, and are referred to as 'B' mice or as 'deprived' mice. Deprived mice can sustain the growth of xenografts of malignant or of normal tissues: thus, human skin and human tumour cells can be grown in 'B' mice which may be regarded as artificial approximations to the genetically thymusless 'nude' mouse.

2. *Corticosteroids.* This category includes a number of natural endogenous corticosteroids, e.g. hydrocortisone (cortisol), testosterone and to a lesser extent corticosterone, but not deoxycorticosterone. In clinical practice the most widely used substances exercising a similar action are prednisone and prednisolone. Cortisol and testosterone respectively may also impair the immune response indirectly by causing a premature involution of the thymuses

of young rodents and in chicks of the *Bursa of Fabricius*. Steroids are most widely used in clinical practice where the intention is to suppress CMI, and it is a remarkable feature of the immunosuppressive steroids that prolonged administration of high doses can suppress or very greatly weaken the reactivity of animals or human beings that have already been sensitized. The organisms most susceptible to the immunosuppressive effects of steroids such as cortisol are those in which there is a relatively low level of endogenous cortisol secretion. Among laboratory animals the most susceptible are rabbits, rats and mice. Inasmuch as injection of unphysiological doses of corticosteroids inhibits their endogenous secretion, it is sometimes advisable to inject ACTH instead, or as well, though unfortunately ACTH cannot stimulate the production of quantities of corticosteroids functionally equivalent to those which may be administered therapeutically.

3. *Antiproliferative agents* are as various as cancer chemotherapeutic agents, from the armoury of which they were, in fact, borrowed. Excluding the ionising irradiations, the principal categories are: nitrogen mustards such as cyclophosphamide, a reminder that mustard gas (sulphur mustard) was one of the first immunosuppressive agents to be discovered; DNA base analogues such as 6-mercaptopurine or its derivative Imuran (azathioprine) and mitotic poisons such as mitomycin and

97

actinomycin-D, which probably act directly upon chromosomes. To these may be added a number of plant alkaloids such as phytopennyblastine and vincomycin with strongly cytotoxic actions.

There is no knowing *a priori* precisely what effect any given antiproliferative agent is going to exercise, but of all of them, as of irradiation, it may be said that there is no evidence of their affecting any distinctively immunological performance of the cell. It is more likely that their immunosuppressive action is achieved by eliminating the proliferative episode that normally accompanies the immune response and is largely responsible for amplifying it from a regional to a body-wide level. It is perhaps of special relevance to this interpretation that excepting antilymphocyte serum (see below) no immunosuppressive agent abolishes the first inflammatory episode of the normal lymphocyte transfer reaction (see page 80). All antiproliferative drugs, however, abolish the later 'flare up' which is probably accompanied by cell division, and might be taken to represent the ampliative element in the normal immunological response.

Although there is no knowing *a priori* what effect any given immunosuppressive agent or procedure will have, empirical evidence shows that at certain dosage levels cyclophosphamide acts as a B-cell inhibitor (see Chapter 2).

4. *Antilymphocyte serum,* by contrast, is predominantly a T-cell inhibitor for it selectively destroys peripheral lymphocytes belonging to the recirculating compartment (Chapter 2); lymphoid cells within lymphoid organs are relatively protected. ALS or the active immunoglobulin-G (ALG) derived from it is prepared by raising a 'heterologous' (xenogeneic) antiserum against lymphocytes of the species in which immunosuppression is to be achieved. Thus an ALS for use in mice is raised by injecting lymphocytes of mice into rabbits, or for use in human beings is raised by injecting human lymphocytes into horses, rabbits, sheep or goats. ALS naturally contains a high concentration of unwanted anti-species antibodies which must be removed by thorough absorption – normally with the red blood corpuscles of the species. Because ALG has a very much lesser effect upon humoral than upon cell mediated immunity, it may be used without the fear that an organism's defences against micro-organisms will be prostrated. The action of ALS is very greatly potentiated by cortisol and also by thymectomy. These combined therapies achieve so high a degree of immunosuppression that even xenotransplantation can be accomplished. Unhappily, ALG is a powerful antigen and anaphylactogen. Even this disability can be partially overcome, however, taking steps to institute a state of immunological tolerance or paralysis with respect to horse serum proteins

before the immunosuppressive treatment begins: treatment with ALG is preceded by intravenous infusions of aggregate-free normal horse IgG (see p. 83).

Intensive immunosuppression is a term that has been used to describe a combination of powerful immunosuppressive procedures used in clinical practice (especially in the treatment of multiple sclerosis). In the most intensive regimen thoracic duct drainage is combined with the administration of ALG and of Imuran and cortisone.

5. *Alloantibody as an immunosuppressive agent.* The inhibition of CMI by homologous humoral antibody is a phenomenon *sui generis*. In the context of transplantation and tumour immunology the phenomenon is known as 'enhancement'. Its effect is to cause transplants of some kinds to survive longer than they otherwise would have done, and to spare both transplanted and autochthonous tumours from some of the consequences of CMI. Enhancement is normally procured either by a passive infusion of antibody of the right specificity or – in those forms of immunity in which both CMI and an antibody response are aroused – by immunizing with antigen treated or administered in such a way that while its capacity to form humoral antibodies is unaffected, the ability to induce CMI is greatly impaired. With ordinary tissue transplants, this is most easily achieved by a pretreatment of the intended recipient of a

graft etc. with lyophilized allogeneic tissue (i.e. tissue dried in the frozen state by sublimation). Antibody-induced immunological suppression is specific in character, but its precise mechanism is unknown. One possibility which has come to be known as 'afferent enhancement' is that the antibody combines with the antigen in such a way as either to divagate it or to impair its antigenicity in some other way. The term 'efferent enhancement', by contrast, is used to describe a state of affairs in which antibody is somehow interposed between a sensitized lymphoid cell and its target, either by acting upon the sensitized lymphoid cell itself or by coating the target cell in such a way that it is no longer recognizable by the aggressor cell, or is in some other way protected from it. There are reasons for believing that antigen-antibody complexes exercise an efficient and specific immunosuppressive action. Indeed, there are encouraging reports that a significant prolongation of life of allografts can be achieved in some species by combining antigenic stimulation with the passive administration of specific antibody. As made clear in the chapter on tolerance (q.v.) it has been suggested that some forms of tolerance are, in reality, the effect of the immunosuppressive action of antigen-antibody complexes. Alloantibody in 'enhancement' may also exercise a *central* inhibitory effect (see Chapter 2) differing from that of other immunosuppressive agents in being antigen-specific in action.

P.B.M.

CHAPTER FOUR
Tumour Immunity

Tumour immunity has been discussed and experimented upon since the early days of the century, but it is only in comparatively recent years that it has been studied in a form which holds out any prospect of clinical usefulness. The concept of tumour immunity arose from the discovery that tumours in mice and rats could sometimes be transplanted from one mouse or rat to another. As a general rule, repeated attempts had to be made before a transplanted tumour line could be established, especially as the mice used (the 'white mouse', the 'grey mouse') were completely heterogeneous in a genetical sense. Nevertheless, a number of rules were established by experimentation: the usual thing was for a tumour first to grow and then to undergo regression, and a mouse in which a tumour had first grown and then dwindled away was absolutely refractory to the growth of that same tumour if it were transplanted on a second occasion. An equally refractory state could sometimes also be brought into being by the inoculation of the intended recipient with normal – particularly embryonic – cells or defibrinated blood. It was to this induced refractory state that Georg Schoene gave the name 'tumour immunity' but early critics, among them Peyton Rous, were not prepared to accept the idea that tumour immunity had any necessary bearing on resistance to autochthonous tumours.*

Rous pointed out that in all probability tumour immunity was not directed against a tumour as a tumour but against a tumour as a foreign or, as we should now say, allogeneic graft. This accusation was all too just, and for very many years the study of tumour immunity turned out to be an enormous red herring, for it was, in effect, the study of transplantation immunity – a subject to which it made important contributions, especially in relation to the genetic background of transplantability (see pp. 74–7).

No further progress in the study of tumour immunity could be made until the development of highly inbred strains of mice at Bar Harbor, Maine, for if a tumour aroused immunity in a mouse belonging to its strain of origin, the immunity could hardly be directed against alloantigens. In this way it came to be discovered that tumours induced in laboratory

---

* Autochthonous means 'springing from the soil in which it lives'. The term 'spontaneous' is not now widely used because it merely signifies our ignorance of causal mechanisms.

animals by carcinogenic chemicals such as 20-methylcholanthrene and oncogenic viruses such as Simian virus (SV) 40 contained distinctive antigens which could arouse transplantation immunity even in the organisms in which the tumours were growing. Among the earlier experiments which demonstrated this phenomenon were those showing that a mouse from which a tumour had been removed, or in which it had been caused to regress by vascular strangulation, was refractory to a further inoculation of the same tumour. Soon afterwards it was shown that even syngeneic mice could be immunized by a prior inoculation of tumour cells.

Though there is an antigenic relationship between tumours aroused by the same oncogenic virus, the antigens that make their appearance in different tumours aroused by the action of methylcholanthrene or other chemical oncogens are not related to each other.

Tumour immunity is in some circumstances a cell mediated immunity of the same general kind as transplantation immunity (Chapter 3).

Immunological surveyance. This affinity between tumour and transplantation immunity led Burnet to propose that the transplantation immunity which prohibits the transplantation of allografts is simply the tiresome by-product of an immunological monitoring system of which the principal teleonomic function is to suppress the growth of tumours.

The immunological surveyance theory has a number of important implications. These are (a) that the 'spontaneous' regression of tumours, instead of being exceptional or a great rarity, must be a not infrequent phenomenon. Indeed, as soon as the possibility of regression became part of the current paradigm, and thus scientifically respectable, reports of regression began to appear with increasing frequency in the medical press. (b) As a corollary of (a), many more tumours must arise in the body than ever became clinically apparent. (c) Procedures likely to affect the body's immunological capability, such as radical and extensive lymphadenectomy, should be embarked upon with great circumspection. The same applies in principle to the use of cancer chemotherapeutic agents which are strongly immunosuppressive in action. A balance must be struck between the direct antitumour effect and the weakening of antitumour immunity. Nevertheless, to reduce the antigenic burden there is a case for the surgical removal of the greater part of a tumour even in the full awareness that the whole tumour cannot be removed. The antigenicity of many autochthonous tumours in experimental animals is well attested, but conclusive evidence of the specific antigenicity to their victims of human tumours is still awaited.

The idea of immunological surveyance is important enough to justify any further energetic trials of its validity. One such trial, the lifelong administration of antilymphocyte serum (p. 99) to CBA mice gave results only partly compatible with the theory, for although the mice were specially vulnerable to polyoma virus, the frequency of tumours not attributable to infection by virus did not increase to the degree which might have been expected if the surveyance theory were unqualifiedly true. Although the CBA strain is one with a naturally low incidence of 'spontaneous' tumours, these experiments on lifelong immunosuppression indicate that the infrequency of tumours in CBA mice is not due to any special vigilance or efficacy of an immunological monitoring system. (For a further discussion of immunological surveyance see Chapter 5.)

Tumour antigens. New antigens that arise in chemically induced tumours have properties *sui generis.* The same applies to tumours raised by physical means such as the implantation of plastic films. The individual specificity of tumour antigens raises special problems from the point of view of treatment, and these problems have not yet been surmounted (but see below: Immunopotentiation).

Enhancement and blocking factors. Like allografts, tumours can excite the formation of humoral antibodies and these bring with them the danger of an interference with CMI leading to a promotion of tumour growth of a kind analogous to 'enhancement' (see p. 100) of normal allografts. It is also possible that tumour immunity is interfered with by the action of 'blocking factors'. Recent research suggests that lymphocytes of tumour-bearing animals or human beings are sometimes hostile towards tumour cells grown in tissue culture, as would be expected if the tumour had aroused some degree of immunity. At the same time, however, it has been reported that the serum of tumour-bearing subjects – particularly those in whom the tumour seems to be growing progressively – also contain a 'blocking factor' which interposes itself between the lymphocytes and what would otherwise be their target, and thus annuls antitumour immunity. Blocking factors are not merely antibodies, but are now thought to be antigen-antibody complexes or even circulating antigens.

Fetal antigens. Among the ideas thrown up by recent cancer research is that tumour neoantigens are 'derepressed' fetal or embryonic antigens, i.e. represent the reawakening of the distinctive and fetal-specific antigenic substances the manufacture of which would normally have been switched off in the course of development. The affinity between *fetal* and *tumour* antigens has been firmly established for cells made malignant by infection with SV40 virus, but evidence relating to other tumours is not yet quite so secure. Inoculation of young fetal cells can nevertheless discourage the growth of tumours induced by methylcholanthrene in mice.

Immunopotentiation

The study of immunopotentiation (the strengthening of the immune response) goes as naturally with the study of tumour immunity as immunosuppression goes with transplantation immunity. If the reasoning in the preceding paragraphs is correct the most effective form of immunopotentiation would be a general strengthening of the cell-mediated arm of the immune response, accompanied if possible by a reduction of humoral immunity. Moreover, immunopotentiation must of necessity be non-specific so as to be effective against all tumour antigens. It is known that bacterial vaccines of micro-organisms such as BCG and of *Corynebacterium parvum* lines elevate antitumour reactivity, and BCG (an attenuated tubercle bacillus) is in quite widespread clinical use already. The most fully worked out example of immunopotentiation in experimental systems, however, is that of the castration of male mice – a procedure which increases to a remarkable degree the resistance of mice to chemically-induced or transplanted syngeneic tumours. Castration, it appears, exercises its immunological effect by retarding the involution of the thymus, increasing the total number rather than the individual reactivity of T cells. These effects are attributed to androgen deprivation in much the same way as the well-known effect of adrenalectomy can be attributed to the withdrawal of the otherwise immunosuppressive action of prednisol or other adrenocortical steroids.

It is unfortunately true to say that in no form of CMI is any immunopotentiating procedure regularly as effective as the heightening of the immune response produced by specific sensitization.

The principal and immediate need is for some systematic investigation of the endocrinological background of immunological control. A beginning has been made with the recognition of a substance 'Thymosin' which expedites the maturation of T cells at least *in vitro.*

Of tumour immunity in general it can, however, be said that the goal of research should be the devising of new means of making use of any immunogenic properties of specific tumour antigens, while at the same time enquiring into and removing the various impediments that prevent tumour immunity from taking its full effect.

P.B.M.

CHAPTER FIVE
Immunological Diseases

Allergy. The most common human disturbance of immunity is allergy. Under this heading comes a wide miscellany of ailments including asthma, hay fever, reactions to foods, cosmetics, animal danders and dust particles, a wide variety of skin afflictions, drug reactions, anaphylactic response serum sickness and allergic responses as an element of many infectious diseases. Some forms of allergy are rather uncommon; for example, fatal reaction following bee sting is rare. On the other hand almost everyone is personally acquainted with a sufferer from hay fever.

Origin of allergy. For the most part allergy is manifest in individuals who are otherwise completely healthy. However, allergy does not arise through any peculiarly 'allergic' property of the antigenic stimulant alone: even an allergen as potent as poison ivy does not cause contact dermatitis in all individuals. Allergy is the response of a susceptible host to repeated

111

exposures to an appropriate antigen. The allergy itself is never manifest at the first contact but only after a state of allergic sensitivity has been aroused. An apparent exception to this rule is that of serum sickness which may follow a single injection of foreign protein (usually horse serum in the form of tetanus antitoxin). However, this paradox is resolved by the fact that the antigen, horse serum protein, enjoys such a long biological half-life in the recipient that sufficient antigen is still present when the primary response has developed.

An explanation of the vulnerability of only some individuals to allergic responses is forthcoming from recent studies of the genetic control of immune responses. Inasmuch as the capacity to respond to particular haptenic configurations is under genetic control, allergic reactivity may be a manifestation of a certain responsive genotype.

Natural role of allergy. What is the natural function of allergy? Is it, as many believe, a protective mechanism gone astray, the price we pay for a hair-trigger sensing system which is fired inappropriately on occasion? We can understand how bronchospasm might be a useful response to an airborne bacterial invader or how the rhinorrhoea characteristic of hay fever could drown an intruding antigen in IgA antibodies, lysozyme and other natural humoral defence factors. Occasionally, however, the cure is worse than the disease. A classic example is provided by lymphocytic choriomeningitis (LCM), a viral infection of mice which is usually associated with severe neurologic damage ending in death. Both humoral immunity and CMI to LCM virus can be recognized, but it appears that the latter response is that which causes the disease, for if cell mediated reactivity to LCM virus is suppressed by antilymphocyte serum then the viraemia is not accompanied by neurological disease.

Tissue damage in allergy. As previously indicated (Chapter 2) the damage to bystander tissue is always a hazard in the nonspecific phase of immunological responses and to some extent allergic tissue damage is the price paid for resisting infection. It is when the response is directed against an antigen treated as if it were a harmful invader that we term the condition an 'allergy'. We have cited an example where cell mediated immunity can cause allergic tissue damage. In humoral immunity, however, tissue damage through immune complex deposition is much more common. The most carefully studied model of this type is chronic serum sickness wherein complexes of foreign serum protein and antibody are deposited in the blood vessel walls and particularly in the vascular endothelium of the renal glomerulus. In these sites they interfere with tissue function both by their physical presence and by the consequences of complement activation and the ensuing inflammation. It is now recognized that this model of immune complex disease very often has a clinical counterpart, especially in chronic viral infection where circulating immune complexes can be easily found. More recently a disease of hitherto unknown etiology, *periarteritis nodosa* in which medium sized blood vessels are disrupted by an inflammatory cell infiltrate, has been attributed to the deposition of immune complexes excited by Australia antigen, the virus of hepatitis.

IgE and immediate allergy. Both humoral and cell mediated immunities may participate in allergy but the special role of IgE in the immediate forms of allergy - those characterized by the abrupt onset of inflammation after contact with antigen - must be emphasized (see also Chapter 1). The role that IgE plays in natural defence is not understood. However, large quantities arise not uncommonly in response to chronic parasitic infections. Mast cells appear to have a receptor for IgE and may therefore become passively armed. Upon contact with antigen, mast cells passively sensitized with IgE release their content of histamine which brings about the vasomotor response characteristic of acute allergy. Susceptibility to allergy of this type can be easily transferred with purified preparations of IgE. However, so far as is known, passive protection against parasitic organisms cannot be conferred in this way.

Treatment of allergy. The manifestations of

allergy are usually treated symptomatically, by using drugs that interfere with the non-specific components of inflammation: for example antihistamines are used in the acute forms of allergy and, in asthma, agents that prevent construction of the bronchioles are very helpful. In the very drastic reaction known as anaphylactic shock large doses of steroid hormones and adrenalin may be required to save life. If the allergen is known it is sometimes possible to 'desensitize' the individual by a protracted schedule of repeated injections of antigen in doses which start at a miniscule level and gradually increase. This is an empirical procedure whose mode of action is poorly understood.

Immunological deficiency. The immunological deficiency diseases are interesting out of proportion to their frequency. They are dramatic because when fully manifest they are incompatible with life and when incomplete are often incompatible with health. Their interest to the immunologist as such lies in what they reveal about the existence and function of human lymphoid subpopulations. A number of these diseases, manifest in the newborn, are known to be genetic in origin and the gene responsible may be either an autosomal or a sex-linked recessive. The classification of immunological deficiency diseases grows ever more complex. However, it is clear that they may be divided into T cell deficiency, B cell deficiency, a mixture of both abnormalities or finally a deficiency in the stem cell population.

The complete syndrome. A child with pure T cell deficiency has its counterpart in the neonatally thymectomized mouse and cannot reject skin allografts or display other features of cell mediated immunity though immunoglobulin function appears normal. On the other hand the agammaglobulinaemic child, with a pure B cell deficiency, is the human analogue of a bursectomized chicken. Such a patient can display CMI including allograft rejection but cannot mount an antibody response. At the moment, apart from the possibility of raising such children in a gnotobiotic environment (an impractical and morally unacceptable procedure), the only hope is to correct the specific defect in immunological performance by transplantation. In agammaglobulinaemia this can be accomplished by passive infusion of immunoglobulins from normal volunteers. Indeed such children are protected initially by the passive infusion of antibody they receive from their mothers. T cell deficiency due to failure of thymic development has been successfully treated by thymic transplantation and in a few cases the severe combined immunodeficiency due to deficient stem cell performance has been successfully treated by the transplantation of bone marrow.

Hypogammaglobulinaemia. Although agammaglobulinaemia is quite rare and

usually fatal in early life, hypogammaglobulinaemia, a relative deficiency of immunoglobulin of varying degrees of severity, is rather
more common. In some forms it is genetic in
origin, but in others it appears to be acquired
often in association with other disease. These
patients are immunologic cripples for they are
susceptible to frequent and exceptionally
severe bacterial infections of both skin and
respiratory tract. Treatment under these
circumstances requires both passive
immunoglobulin and antibiosis.

The frequency of a relative deficiency of T
cell function and its manifestations are not
known. Until recently there was no convenient
way to assess relative T cell function, but with
the advent of *in vitro* analysis of response to
mitogens specific for T cells it has become
possible to screen patients for their presence.
It is interesting that in advanced malignancy,
chronic inflammatory bowel disease and
rheumatoid arthritis a relative deficiency of T
cell response has been discovered both by *in
vitro* criteria and by skin tests for delayed
hypersensitivity. Whether deficiency and
disease are cause or effect and what role
deficiency plays in the manifestations
associated with these disease states are at
present conjectural.

A type of acquired immunologic deficiency
that is growing more common is that depression of function which results from the use of
immunosuppressive agents. For example

patients with renal transplants are at present more likely to die as a result of overwhelming infection than from rejection of their allografts.

Consequences of pregnancy. The immunological relationship between mother and developing fetus is unique, for considered as a natural allograft the fetus is usually tolerated without danger to either party. However, matters occasionally miscarry.

Rh disease. One rather common misadventure is the condition known as erythroblastosis fetalis which occurs under the following circumstances. The separation of the maternal and fetal blood streams *in utero* is occasionally imperfect during the latter months of pregnancy and during parturition there is an additional opportunity for fetal blood to escape into the mother. If the mother is Rh negative, i.e. lacks a principal erythrocyte antigen of the rhesus series and the child is Rh positive (because the father was so) then the mother may become immunized. As this event usually occurs very late in pregnancy the first child of Rh-incompatible parents is usually unaffected. A second such pregnancy will however occur in an already sensitized mother and hence small leakages of erythrocyte antigen will result in a considerable antibody response, in the course of which antibodies, particularly of the IgG class, will enter the fetal circulation where opsonization of fetal erythrocytes will occur and eventually cause their destruction. If such an event occurs early in pregnancy the child may be stillborn. If the maternal antibodies enter the fetus relatively late in pregnancy the child may appear normal on birth but develops an extreme anaemia and jaundice during the first twenty-four hours of life. This in turn may either kill the child or produce severe damage to the central nervous system.

Treatment of haemolytic disease. Until very recently the accepted treatment of newborns imperilled by haemolytic disease was exchange transfusion. However this could only deal with the problems arising after birth and was not without complications of its own. A particularly instructive example of the application of basic immunology to clinical treatment is embodied in the modern treatment of this condition. When Rh incompatibility is known to exist, the mother can be treated by passive infusion of high titre anti-Rh serum at the time of parturition. This serum will mop up any Rh positive fetal erythrocytes in the maternal circulation and thus prevent an immune response by the mother; in addition it may diminish her response by an inhibitory process which takes advantage of the negative feedback principle referred to on p. 52.

Damages to the mother. One of the adaptations which makes possible the growth of the fetal allograft is a state of decreased immune reactivity towards paternal antigens perhaps akin to the blocking phenomenon referred to in other contexts (pp. 100 and 108), and this in conjunction with the lack of expression of histocompatibility antigens in the cytotrophoblast is usually adequate to prevent an immune response on the part of the mother. This arrangement is not entirely without its dangers to the mother, for occasionally bits of placenta are left behind which persist as benign growths known as 'moles' which must be surgically removed. On rare occasions things go one step further and persistent placental elements give rise to a malignant growth known as a chorioepithelioma. Although paternal, i.e. allograft, antigens are contained within the tumour, the state of specific immunologic depression induced by the pregnancy in the mother makes her unable to reject this otherwise highly antigenic tumour. The cytotoxic drug methotrexate (amethopterin: a folic acid antagonist) has been extremely successful in its treatment. The accepted reason for its success is that it prevents the tumour from dividing until the mother recovers her immunological reactivity. Another hypothetical possibility is that methotrexate also contributes by suppressing the humoral immune response of the mother thereby removing or reducing blocking antibody and potentiating T cell reactivity.

Autoimmune diseases. A large group of poorly understood diseases is attributed to autoimmunity. It has become fashionable to speculate upon an autoimmune origin of disease whenever pathogenesis and aetiology are obscure. It is probable that the great majority of these are not autoimmune in the sense with which the word is usually used but in order to understand this category of disease we must return to the concept of *self tolerance.*

Self tolerance. It was Ehrlich in the nineteenth century who first used the notion of a *horror autotoxicus* to explain the fact that the destructive potential of phagocytes was not ordinarily exercised against other tissues of the same organism. Burnet, while propounding the theory of somatic mutation (p. 105) to explain the diversity of lymphocyte reactivities, realized that he would have to include in his general theory a mechanism for eliminating lymphocyte lineages of self-reactive potential – 'forbidden clones'. The simplest regulating device would make use of antigen itself. If, during differentiation, lymphocytes with receptors for antigen in their immediate environment were to be destroyed, the repertoire of each organism would be complete except for reactions to the antigens it possessed itself. This concept was regarded as confirmed when it came to be shown that the introduction of antigen into animals undergoing immunologic maturation resulted in tolerance towards that antigen (see pp. 83-93). These notions were formulated before the discovery of the clear distinction between B and T cells and their different properties.

Tolerance in T and B cells. It now appears that B and T cells differ in the requirements for both the induction and maintenance of tolerance. T cells can become tolerant when exposed to relatively low concentrations of antigen and tolerance is long lasting both because the dosage threshold of induction is low and because the turnover rate of T lymphocytes is slow. B cells on the other hand require high concentrations of antigens for tolerance induction and because they have a high threshold and a more rapid turnover rate tolerance is more difficult to maintain. The possibility must now therefore be entertained that there may exist in perfectly normal individuals B cells not tolerant of self antigens because concentration of these antigens in the milieu of the lymphocyte is too low. Under ordinary circumstances such non-tolerant cells may still not mount an immune response against these antigens for a variety of reasons: the antigens in their native form may be relatively or totally non-immunogenic, or they may be thymus-dependent antigens so that in the absence of reactive T cells immunization will not occur or be sustained; or finally the concentration of antigen may be too low for immunization as well as for tolerance induction. (The evidence that such B cells exist is suggested by the occurrence of antigen binding of self proteins by lymphocytes in normal animals and humans.)

Origin of autoimmunity. We are now in a position to examine the ways in which autoimmune disease could theoretically arise.

1. One such way is an exposure to antigen from a privileged site, i.e. a site in which it could not normally have aroused immunity. A good example here is *sympathetic ophthalmia* in which, after a penetrating injury to one eye, the undamaged eye undergoes violent inflammatory destruction of the retina which develops within a week or two of the original injury. As the eye like the central nervous system (of which it is embryologically a part) is a privileged site, the antigens of the retina are not ordinarily available for tolerance induction or maintenance.

2. A second way in which 'autoimmune' reactions might be aroused is through an alteration in the physical or chemical form of self antigens as a result of aggregation or denaturation or coupling to some external agent such as a drug. Under these circumstances determinants which were previously hidden or exposed determinants which are now modified can be recognized as foreign and a reaction against them undertaken. For example it is well known that in thermal burns there is often the transient appearance of antibodies that react with native skin. It is likely that under these circumstances a heat

denaturation of skin components triggers the response.

3. A third way in which an autoimmune response might theoretically occur would be if antigen ordinarily present below both the thresholds for tolerance or immunization were suddenly to increase in concentration as a result of disease or injury. Thus if injury to the thyroid gland caused thyroglobulin in the circulation to exceed the immunization threshold then a reaction could occur.

4. Similarly the introduction into the body of foreign antigens which are closely related to self antigens may cause the production of *cross reacting* antibodies or may bypass the T cell, which is tolererant, and trigger the B cell directly. Recent experiments have shown extensive cross reactivity between cell surface histocompatibility antigens, renal basement membranal antigens and bacterial antigens, and these studies suggest that exposure to exogenous bacterial antigens has considerable potential to bring about host tissue damage.

5. *Viral cell surface antigen.* Probably one of the most important mechanisms that may arouse a self-destructive reaction is the infection of a body cell by a virus or other micro-organism which expresses a portion of its distinctive surface or capsular antigen on the surface of the infected cell. Under these circumstances reactivity to the foreign antigens of the infective agent directed against the site of expression necessarily brings about destruc-

tion of the infected host cell as well. It is now clear that a number of common viral infections have these properties. Indeed in a large number of chronic inflammatory diseases thought at the moment to be autoimmune, an unrecognized infectious agent may, in fact, be responsible for triggering and maintaining the process.

The expression of the foreign antigens of an infectious agent on the cell surface or indeed the coupling of any foreign material to the cell surface, e.g. the binding of a drug, is yet another mechanism through which autoimmune disease might be aroused. These antigens might act as T cell stimulants and therefore act as a kind of carrier to promote the reaction of B cells to adjacent self antigen determinants.

Appropriate experimental models can be adduced as evidence to incriminate all the above mentioned possibilities as causes of autoimmune tissue damage. An important point about all these processes is that they occur in the presence of a normal immunological response. The manifestations of autoimmunity depend upon the peculiar circumstances involved and not upon a diseased state of the immunological response system.

6. *The forbidden clone.* One theoretical mechanism not yet mentioned which might be considered an archetypal cause of autoimmune disease is the generation of a forbidden autoreactive clone. Whether this ever occurs

naturally and, if it does so, how often, is at present entirely unknown. In the laboratory it is possible to demonstrate B cells that can bind some self antigens. As already explained above, the presence of such cells is not necessarily ominous. Under highly contrived experimental circumstances it is possible to provoke the formation of T cells which have syngeneic reactivity. However, these experiments are too recent for confident evaluation.

Autoantibody. Autoantibodies may be found in normal, healthy people with a frequency and in a variety that increases as the search for them becomes more intense. It is quite clear that small amounts of these autoantibodies can occur in completely healthy individuals with no apparent untoward consequences. The frequency of autoantibody detected and their titre tends to rise as the population ages. The significance of this presence is not understood. However, it is possible that these antibodies serve a natural role in the catabolism of self components.

Under normal circumstances T cell reactivity is not demonstrable. However, it remains possible that the elaboration of autoantibody is regulated by T cells and that autoimmunity, i.e. the secretion of inappropriate antibodies, or their secretion in vastly increased amounts, can come about through the breakdown of a controlling mechanism.

Criteria for autoimmunity. The usual criteria used to assign a given condition to autoimmunity include the histopathological appearances, the presence of autoantibodies, the presence of self-reactive cell mediated immunity, a therapeutic response to anti-inflammatory or immunosuppressive drugs, and the absence of any other reasonable cause. The finding of an inflammatory infiltrate consisting of lymphocytes, plasma cells and macrophages is compatible with autoimmune disease. However, such granulomas are also to be found in chronic infection and trauma. Autoantibodies, as we have noted, are often present in normal individuals and only high titres need justifiably raise suspicion. The presence of self-reactive T cells has been difficult to demonstrate even in the laboratory. This criterion may become more useful as *in vitro* assays for T cell function become more refined. The response to anti-inflammatory and/or immunosuppressive drugs is clearly not diagnostic, and most often disease is attributed to autoimmunity because of a conjunction of compatible findings when there is no other obvious cause.

Animal models of autoimmunity. A large number of autoimmune diseases have been produced in the laboratory by mixing tissue homogenates or tissue extracts with an adjuvant – usually Freund's complete adjuvant (p. 3) – and injecting this mixture into suitable recipients. In these circumstances a single immunization will often suffice to produce disease, and by choosing the tissue antigen beforehand the site of disease can be chosen in advance. Therefore there are well described models of thyroiditis, orchitis, adrenalitis, encephalomyelitis and so forth. Not all strains of animals, however, are equally susceptible to the induction of autoimmune disease by this process. It is known that the susceptibility to autoimmune thyroiditis is genetically controlled in the chicken and it is well known that susceptibility to adjuvant arthritis in rats varies from strain to strain.

Role of CMI and humoral immunity. In experimental autoimmune disease both cell mediated immunity and autoantibody formation are aroused, and their relative roles in autoimmune tissue damage have been the subject of much controversy. A method that has been useful in assessing the relative importance of CMI and HI has been to see whether the disease can be transferred to a second host either by the passive infusion of antibody or by the adoptive transfer of immunized cells. Under these circumstances it is usually observed that the disease can be transferred with cells but not with serum. However, the antibodies still probably play a pathogenic role, for the complete histological picture is best reproduced in the secondary hosts by the combination of cells and antibody. An extremely interesting form of autoimmune disease occurs spontaneously in the NZB (New Zealand Black) mouse. Born healthy, these mice develop at about three months of age a complex of autoimmune manifestations. These are rather similar to the human disease lupus erythematosus. The findings include antibody-mediated haemolytic anaemia, nephritis, the presence of LE cells and of many autoantibodies, an aberration of immune function with T cell deficiency and, often late in the course of the disease, lymphoma. It now seems likely that many of the manifestations of this process can be explained by the interaction of chronic viral infection, and genetically determined limitations of immune responsiveness. The findings in this model have had considerable influence on thought about clinical autoimmunity, and have stimulated the search for similar features in human disease.

Human autoimmune disease ranges from conditions in which autoimmune processes are clearly implicated to those in which it is extremely dubious. Amongst the former are the antibody-mediated haemolytic anaemias. Autohaemagglutinins and autohaemolysins arise not infrequently after exposure to a number of drugs and chemicals in many disease states such as the leukaemias, and in association with acute infection.

Under these circumstances destruction of the red cells is clearly the direct consequence of autoantibody attachment. Thyroiditis is another relatively clear-cut example of autoimmune disease in man. Here the manifestations bear a striking resemblance to the experimental model, with high titres of antibodies to thyroglobulin, the presence of a chronic inflammatory infiltrate into the thyroid gland resembling very much the allograft response, and ultimately interference with thyroid gland function. Lupus erythematosus (already mentioned) is a disease which affects young females predominantly, and is characterized by widespread tissue involvement, high titres of autoantibodies, immune complex deposition and aberration of immunologic function. In these examples autoimmune manifestations are prominent and play a definite role in the state of ill health which follows. However, it now appears more likely that the trigger for autoimmune pathogenesis is an external stimulus, e.g. a persistent infection, rather than the development of forbidden reactive clones. For example, it is now thought likely that the condition known as subacute sclerosing panencephalomyelitis (SSPE) is due to chronic persistence of measles virus. Before the identification of this virus such an illness might well have passed for a 'spontaneous' autoimmune disease.

Possible autoimmune diseases. There is a large variety of diseases in which it is possible that autoimmune mechanisms play a role. Amongst these are such conditions as rheumatoid arthritis in which the presence of autoantibody, a compatible histology, and response to drugs are suggestive. Another candidate is disseminated sclerosis, which bears a superficial resemblance to the animal models of allergic encephalomyelitis. The role of genetic factors, especially those that influence immune responsiveness, is suggested by the occasionally strong family history of autoimmune disease and by the tendency for patients with one kind of autoimmune disease to be more likely to develop a second. A very striking recent finding has been the almost universal association of ankylosing spondylitis (a variant within the rheumatoid arthritis family) with a particular histocompatibility antigen. In view of what is known about the linkage between immune response and histocompatibility genes in animals, this association strongly suggests that similar mechanisms are at work.

Summary

A large and miscellaneous group of human diseases have been loosely described as autoimmune in origin. The etiology and pathogenesis of these diseases is often not clear, but what is clear is that autoantibodies in high titre are often found which in some cases may be the direct cause of severe tissue damage. Evidence of cell mediated autoimmunity is less compelling at the moment, but this may be due to technical difficulties of recognition. There is at the moment no direct evidence to suggest a role for forbidden clones of autoreactive lymphocytes or for theories which rest upon failures of immunological regulation.

The most attractive theory is that most, if not all of these ailments arise in normally responsive individuals. The trigger may be an infection or some other agent which modifies the cell surface, causes the release of antigen from privileged sites or raises the normal concentration of antigen to the immunizing threshold. Important modifying host factors, such as genetic susceptibility or genetic immunological capacity, which turn what might otherwise be an acute self-limited process into a chronic tissue-damaging process, also require consideration. It should be pointed out that the failure to culture an organism from the tissues of individuals with such diseases in which a virus etiology is suspected does not disprove its complicity in the disease process, for there are a number of well-known animal models in which attempted cultivation also fails.

Moreover it is important to re-emphasize that tissue damage under these circumstances may be the direct consequence of humoral immunity or CMI, or could represent the action of normal reparative processes that lead to the destruction of infected or otherwise damaged tissue. Another possibility is that it might represent the 'innocent bystander' effect referred to on pp. 61 and 113.

Malignancy. Malfunction of the immune response has also been implicated in malignancy. Under this heading we can consider malignancies which arise from cells of the immune system directly. Included amongst these are the lymphomas, the reticulum cell sarcomas, Hodgkin's disease and the myelomata. Apart from the general interest in these tumours from an oncological point of view, some features are of particular interest to the immunologist. For example, aberrations of immune function are often associated even with early forms of these malignancies. Thus, for example, defective cell mediated immunity is characteristic of Hodgkin's disease. The cellular origin of these tumours is in some cases obvious as, for example, in the myeloma which derives from a plasma cell. However, the detailed classification of the lymphomas is only just becoming possible as reagents which characterize the distinctive differentiation antigens of these cells are becoming available. In this respect it is interesting that most chronic lymphatic leukaemias in man appear to be of B cell origin.

Immune surveyance. One of the natural functions which has been ascribed to the immune system is that of surveyance against the development of malignant clones of cells. This extremely attractive theory, for which there is a good deal of circumstantial evidence, states that lymphocytes, more particularly recirculating T lymphocytes, are programmed to distinguish between self antigens and foreign antigens. When a neoplastic cell arises, it expresses tumour specific antigens which are recognized as foreign and can therefore become the subject of an immune attack which eliminates the abnormal cell and its progeny. Corroborating this hypothesis experimentally has been difficult, and certain interesting experimental findings reveal the limitations of the hypothesis of immune surveyance. Mice continuously immunosuppressed from birth did not show any increment in naturally occurring malignancy when compared with the incidence in appropriate controls. On the other hand, such animals were more susceptible to viral oncogenesis (see also p. 107). The most extensive information relevant to man comes from a study of patients bearing renal allografts. These patients, often treated with immunosuppressive agents in high doses and for long periods of time, develop malignant disease much more often than the population from which they are drawn. However, the type of malignancy that occurs is not simply a general scaling up of the incidence of the disease in the community: approximately 50% are lymphomas or reticulum cell sarcomas, and tumours in rare sites such as the intra-cranial cavity were inexplicably common. Recent studies have emphasized that tumours may also arise in situations of chronic low grade immune stimulation, especially when combined with immunosuppression; for example, the combination of repeated casein immunization and the administration of cytotoxic drugs produces a high incidence of tumours, and so does chronic low grade graft-versus-host disease (pp. 79-86). Moreover, we have already mentioned that NZB mice often die from lymphomatous tumours. It may well be that immunosuppression, i.e. the absence of immune surveyance, is a necessary but not sufficient cause of malignancy, and that some second factor, such as an oncogenic virus, a mutagenic stimulus, ionising irradiation, or chronic immune stimulation, is also required. Chronic immune stimulation may play an indirect role inasmuch as blast cells are more susceptible to certain virus infections, and moreover the process of cell division may derepress latent viral genomes residing in the cell.

Ageing. Finally, a failure of immunologic function may be related to the process of ageing. Lymphocytes were formerly believed to exert a trephocytic function, i.e. to be a mobile squad of mechanics that serviced the tissues and kept them in good order. If indeed one of their functions were the destruction and elimination of defective cells (and we have already indicated that the natural function of autoantibody might be to enhance the catabolism of tissue breakdown products), then a failure of this system could lead to progressive tissue and organ malfunction, increase susceptibility to disease, decrease ability to repair etc., i.e. all those characteristics which combine to produce the syndrome of a senescent individual. The fact that immunologic function changes in the ageing organism is now quite well documented in a wide variety of animal species, including man. The decline in T cell function and perhaps T cell control with increasing age is particularly evident, and quite an attractive theory of ageing has already been built upon these and other pieces of evidence of similar data. A major difficulty is that of distinguishing cause from effect, for if malfunction of the immune system is used to explain secondary failures in other tissues, we are still left with the problem of accounting for the primary failure itself.

Afterword

In spite of its spectacularly rapid progress immunology still abounds with unsolved problems and with problem areas not yet fully explored. This is a sign of vitality rather than a reason for regret.

Among the particular questions raised in the foregoing text have been these: is there such a phenomenon as low zone tolerance in transplantation systems? Is tolerance a state of essential non-reactivity or is it actively maintained by, for example, the action of suppressor T cells? Are there or are there not such things as tolerant *cells*? Does the information which underwrites the synthesis of antibodies arise mutationally in the cell lineage of which the end products are lymphocytes, or does it reside in the zygote? Do human tumours possess specific antigens and if so can this property be put to use therapeutically?

Among the problem areas in need of further exploration are: the functional taxonomy of

137

lymphocytes, the endocrine control of the immune response, immunopotentiation generally, the complete elucidation of the nature and mode of action of transfer factor and the relevance of HLA type to susceptibility to disease.

Research needed to answer these questions or open up these subject areas is of the kind the critics ignorant of the scientific process often describe as 'academic'. The pejorative use of the word 'academic' is a philosophical bêtise that instantly identifies the man of little learning.

The backwardness and snail-like progress of immunology from the days of Bordet until the mid-'thirties should be warning enough against the dangers of abandoning what Bacon called *experiments of light* for research dedicated to the policy of quick returns.

Glossary

The following glossary explains the technical terms used in this book. Cross references are italicized.

ADJUVANT, ADJUVANTICITY Some *antigens* in some animals – e.g. purified bovine gamma globulin in mice – will not excite immunity unless they are administered with substances of the class known as adjuvants. The property of conferring immunogenicity on an antigen that might not otherwise be immunogenic is sometimes referred to as 'adjuvanticity', which may be an intrinsic property of the antigenic substance. Adjuvants are also regularly used to potentiate immune responses.

ALLERGY Form of *hypersensitivity* of unknown functional significance, marked by deleterious and exaggerated responses to *antigens* such as pollen or house dust, wool, hair, fur or skin scales (danders), and other

139

substances that are not intrinsically noxious. Allergic reactivity can be passively transferred by certain antibodies often called 'reagins'. The most effective are of class IgE because their special structure enables them to bind to the surface of mast cells and circulating basophils; these cells lose their granular structure and release vasoactive amines that are the immediate cause of *anaphylaxis* or allergic reactivity.

ALLOANTIGENS Any antigen that distinguishes one member of a species from another, but especially an 'allograft' from its recipient.

ALLOGRAFT A graft transplanted to another genetically distinct member of the same species, hence 'allogeneic' transplantation, e.g. grafts from mouse to mouse or man to man.

ALLOTYPE Antibodies, like many other macromolecules in the body, exist in variant forms that enjoy a stable and genetically enforced partition among the members of a population (polymorphism). Polymorphic variants of antibodies are referred to as allotypes, and allotypic differences are inherited according to straightforward Mendelian rules.

ANAMNESTIC RESPONSE See PRIMARY RESPONSE.

ANAPHYLAXIS Literally the opposite of *prophylaxis*, and refers to a deleterious rather than protective response to an antigen, e.g. of *hypersensitivity*, and of no apparent functional significance. Some animals – especially guinea pigs, dogs and human beings – are especially susceptible to anaphylactic shock, for the systemic administration of *antigen* to an already immunized subject leads to widespread edema, respiratory distress and, in extreme cases, heart failure and death. Anaphylactic shock is mediated through the action of histamine. Animals such as mice that are resistant to the action of histamine are proportionately resistant to anaphylactic shock.

ANTIBODY Blood protein, invariably an *immunoglobulin* that is the agent of *humoral immunity*. See Chapter 1 and Table 3, p. 37, for the different varieties of immunoglobulin. See also *idiotype, allotype*.

ANTIGEN An agent that excites an immunological response whether of *immunity, tolerance* or *sensitivity*. See also *immunogen, tolerogen, hapten*.

ARTHUS REACTION The acute local inflammation associated with the congregation of polymorphs and sometimes leading to tissue death which in some animals, especially rabbits, accompanies the meeting of *antigen* with *antibody* within the tissues. The antigen-antibody complexes bind and activate complement. Elements of complement are liberated that attract polymorphs and set up the erythema and edema characteristic of inflammation. 'Farmer's lung' is a hypersensitivity of the Arthus type excited by fungal antigens in mouldy hay.

AUTOGRAFT A graft transplanted from one part to another on the same individual.

B CELL See LYMPHOCYTE.

BLAST CELL The suffix 'blast' is often used to distinguish a progenitor cell from a mature cell distinguished by the suffix '-cyte' – e.g. lymphoblast, lymphocyte; myeloblast, myelocyte. In the context of *MLR* a blast cell refers to a lymphoid cell which has enlarged and started to synthesize DNA in preparation for cell division. The formation of blast cells is usually recognized by their uptake of, for example, tritiated thymidine.

BURSA OF FABRICIUS An organ arising as a diverticulum from the hind end of the gut of birds which has no exact anatomical analogue in mammals. The bursa acts towards *B cells* as the thymus towards *T cells*. The bone marrow in mammals is thought to be functionally the equivalent of the bursa, so that the designation 'B cell' is equally valid for mammals and birds.

CARRIER See HAPTEN.

CLONE The entire population of cells, in theory genetically identical, that have been derived by mitotic division from a single progenitor. Thus antibodies are said to be monoclonal when produced by the descendants of a single cell.

COMPLEMENT A complex of blood-borne reagents that bring about the lysis of cells in association with antibody directed against them. The nine protein components are

142

activated in sequence to form a cascade of enzymes. Each, once activated, potentiates the effects of the next in the series. The last components cause membrane damage and cell death. Earlier components (C3) promote phagocytosis by macrophages and polymorphs.

The complement sequence can be activated either by binding to antigen/antibody complexes (the 'classical' pathway) or by extrinsic agents such as endotoxin, and also by complement fragments – the alternate (*sic*) pathway. The binding of complement by immune complexes (complement fixation) is sometimes the only method by which an antigen/antibody reaction can be known to have taken place.

In the very old literature complement may be referred to as 'alexin' or as 'amboceptor'.

DETERMINANT GROUP (= EPITOPE) The particular molecular configuration in the molecule of an *immunogen* which confers specificity on the immune response and against which immunity is primarily directed.

DIALYSIS Ultrafiltration by diffusion through a cellulose nitrate membrane. Dialysis normally retains soluble proteins but not oligosaccharides, oligopeptides and oligonucleotides, i.e. molecules smaller than proteins.

ELECTROPHORESIS The separation of soluble macromolecules in a potential gradient by reason of differences of electrical charge.

ENHANCEMENT In the context of organ

An Introduction to Immunology

transplantation, enhancement refers to the state of specific non-reactivity akin to, but distinct from *tolerance* brought about by the action of circulating *antibody*. Like *immunity*, enhancement may be passively transferred from one animal to another or may be actively acquired.

EPITOPE See DETERMINANT GROUP.

GAMMAGLOBULIN Historically this term describes the component of serum globulins which contains most of the antibody. *Immunoglobulin* is now more commonly used. The serum globulins generally (γ , β , and α_1 and α_2) are characterized by their electrophoretic mobility.

H-2 COMPLEX See MHC.

HLA COMPLEX See MHC.

HAPLOTYPE The complement of *histocompatibility antigens* found on one chromosome of a pair and therefore – barring crossing over – inherited *en bloc*.

HAPTEN When the *determinant group* of an *immunogen* exists as a molecule in its own right, it is referred to as a hapten. An example is dinitrophenol (DNP), the conjugation of which with protein may arouse an immunity directed specifically against DNP. The body of the antigen molecule other than the determinant group is referred to as the 'carrier'. Carrier and determinant group may both be antigenic.

HISTOCOMPATIBILITY GENES The genes responsible for *alloantigenic differences*. In

144

most animals evolution has taken such a course that the major histocompatibility genes are situated on a chromosome stretch known as *major histocompatibility complex* (MHC, *q.v.*).

HUMORAL IMMUNITY Form of immunity that is mediated through the action of soluble blood-borne substances, especially *antibodies, complement.*

HYPERSENSITIVITY Form of reactivity towards *antigen* that is marked by deleterious and functionally extravagant local or systemic actions. The hypersensitivities include the *Arthus Reaction, allergy, anaphylaxis* and *immediate* and '*delayed*' types of *hypersensitivity.*

HYPERSENSITIVITY, DELAYED The local reactivity to antigen that usually accompanies *cell mediated immunity.* In this form of hypersensitivity the introduction of antigen into the skin – e.g. of tuberculin into the skin of patients with an active or former tubercular infection – is followed by the relatively slow (5-24 hours) development of reddening, edema and hardening of the skin, accompanied by the infiltration of lymphocytes into the tissues. *Cell mediated immunities* in general can be made to perform as delayed type hypersensitivity reactions.

HYPERSENSITIVITY, IMMEDIATE A form of local hyperreactivity to antigen associated with *humoral immunity.* Its manifestations include (a) the *Arthus Reaction,* (b) the 'wheal and flare' reaction mediated through allergic antibodies (reagins).

IDIOTYPE An *antibody* to a newly introduced *immunogen* is itself a protein new to the body and as such can be antigenic. The same applies to any antibody that may be manufactured against it. The theory that immunological regulation in an individual is secured by a multiple interaction between antibodies, anti-antibodies and anti-anti-antibodies is sometimes known as 'network theory'. The structural characteristic that confers antigenicity upon an antibody and differentiates it from antibodies to other antigens is referred to as its 'idiotype'. The idiotype determinant is on the variable (V) region of the antibody molecule (see Fig. 1), where antibody combines with its antigen.

IMMUNITY State entered into as a consequence of exposure to an *immunogen*, the effect of which is to destroy, sequester, inactivate or otherwise annul the action of an *antigen* or its vehicle. See also *humoral immunity, cell mediated immunity, hypersensitivity.*

IMMUNITY, ACTIVELY ACQUIRED Immune state entered into as a consequence of an organism's own exposure to an *immunogen.*

IMMUNITY, ADOPTIVE Immunity brought into being by the introduction into the subject not of antisera, but of specifically sensitized cells, usually of the lymphoid family. Adoptive immunity is thus to *cell mediated immunity* what passive immunity is to *humoral immunity*. Adoptively immunized animals behave like actively immunized animals in respect of the duration of immunity and the response to renewed confrontation with antigen. Adoptive immunization can be carried out only when the recipient is so treated or so related to the donor that the adoptively transferred cells are not destroyed as *allografts*; but see *transfer factor*. *Humoral* as well as cell mediated immunity may be acquired by cell transfer.

IMMUNITY, CELL MEDIATED Form of immunity mediated through the action of sensitized blood-borne cells, especially those of the lymphoid system.

IMMUNITY, PASSIVELY ACQUIRED Immune state acquired at second hand by the introduction of antibody-containing serum from a donor that has been actively immunized. Examples are the prophylactic or therapeutic use of antitoxic sera prepared by the active immunization of horses, or alternatively the transfusion of sera containing anti-bacterial or anti-viral antibodies from convalescent patients. The fetuses of amniote animals acquire immunity passively from the mother through the yolk sac, chorioallantoic placenta or the first milk, 'colostrum'.

IMMUNODIFFUSION The procedure in which soluble antigens and their corresponding antibodies are allowed to diffuse towards each other in an agar or gelatin gel so that the two reagents confront each other over a wide range of concentrations. The reagents interact at their optimum concentrations to form a visible precipitate or band in the gel. When several antigens diffuse towards their corresponding antibodies, several bands of precipitation will appear where each antigen antibody system reaches its optimum concentration. This makes it possible for a mixture of antigens to be separated and identified.

IMMUNOELECTROPHORESIS A combination of *electrophoresis* and *immunodiffusion* which makes it possible for immunological reagents to be distinguished by differences both of electric charge and of diffusivity.

IMMUNOGEN An antigen administered in such a form or such a way that it excites *immunity* or *sensitivity* rather than, for example, *tolerance*.

IMMUNOGLOBULIN (Ig) Functionally and structurally differentiated classes of globulins that act as antibodies. See Chapter 1 and Table 3, p. 37.

IMMUNOLOGICAL SURVEYANCE (=IMMUNOLOGICAL SURVEILLANCE) The theory that the form of immunological reactivity of which *allograft* rejection is the principal manifestation has as its principal and primary function the detection and eradication of cells that have undergone a malignant transformation, e.g. by the action of a virus or chemical oncogen.

IMMUNOLOGICALLY COMPETENT CELL

Term coined to distinguish immunological capability from immunological performance, so distinguishing a 'virgin' lymphocyte from a lymphocyte already engaged by antigen. With newer knowledge of the degree of cellular co-operation in the immune response, the term is falling out of use, but it is still widely found in older literature.

IMMUNOPOTENTIATION The augmentation of the immunoligical response, and thus the opposite of *immunosuppression.*

IMMUNOSUPPRESSION Diminution of *immunity* by the use of, for example, ionising radiations, radiomimetic drugs such as the alkylating agents, and anti-proliferative agents such as the nucleic acid base analogues, e.g. mercaptopurine. Steroids of the cortisone family are also immunosuppressive.

LYMPHOCYTE Member of the family of blood-borne cells that is principally responsible for the transaction of immunological responses. Subdivided into B cells, the agents of humoral immunity, T cells, the agents of *cell mediated immunity*, and a small proportion of other lymphoid cells including K (= killer) cells and 'null' cells that perform special immunological functions.

MHC The chromosomal region containing the major *histocompatibility genes* of a species. In mice, the H2 gene complex is the MHC. In other organisms, because they must of necessity be recognized on leucocytes, the MHC is recognized by the suffix LA. Thus the

MHC of man is HLA (short for human leucocyte antigen) and in dogs is DLA.

MLC = MIXED LYMPHOCYTE CULTURE See MLR.

MLR (= MIXED LYMPHOCYTE REACTION) Reaction to an *alloantigen in vitro* made possible by confronting the lymphocytes of one individual with lymphocytes or other antigenic cells from a member of the same species in a 'mixed lymphocyte culture.' Under appropriate culture conditions mixed lymphocyte reactions can also occur to xenoantigens. The reaction is marked by the formation of *blast cells* usually followed by proliferation.

NETWORK THEORY See IDIOTYPE.

PARALYSIS Is sometimes used interchangeably with tolerance, but is often used rather specially with reference to soluble antigens where tolerance would be used in the context of transplantation.

PRIMARY RESPONSE An animal's response to its first confrontation with an *immunogen*, distinguished from the secondary, 'anamnestic' response, the more powerful response of quicker onset which often follows a second exposure to immunogen.

PROPHYLAXIS A protective immunization to enhance *active immunity* by in effect converting a *primary* into a *secondary* response or by providing ready-made the antibodies that would normally be formed only in *active immunity*. Examples are vaccination by *attenuated* or inactivated viral and bacterial vaccines or by detoxified toxins (toxoids).

SECONDARY RESPONSE See PRIMARY RESPONSE.

SEROLOGY That part of immunology which has to do specially with the recognition of *antigens* by using *antibodies* as reagents.

SYNGENEIC Having as nearly as possible the same genetic constitution. Identical twins are syngeneic, and so also to a close approximation, are members of highly inbred strains of mice, differences of sex apart.

SYNGENESIO-TRANSPLANT Found in older literature to refer to grafts transplanted between animals enjoying a family, though not necessarily a genetic, relationship – e.g. grafts between sibs. Superseded now by *syngeneic*.

T CELL See LYMPHOCYTE.

T LOCUS A chromosomal stretch recognizable in embryonic mice by reason of the fact that some mutant T alleles cause deformities in the formation of the tail and the hind end of the embryonic axis generally. Genes of the T locus determine antigenic differences that can be recognized by orthodox serological methods. The T locus in mice has been described as the embryonic analogue of the *MHC* of adults.

TOLERANCE (=PARALYSIS, IMMU-NOLOGICAL) State of specific non-reactivity towards an *antigen* that might otherwise have aroused some form of immunity. Fully tolerant animals treat antigens as native substances. Animals which do not respond to antigens because of *immunosuppression* or for genetic reasons are not normally referred to as tolerant. See also *enhancement, immunosuppression.*

TOLEROGEN *Antigen* administered in a form or in a way that it confers *tolerance* rather than *immunity.*

TRANSFER FACTOR An agent of unknown composition that makes possible the transfer of *cell mediated immunity* under conditions in which living leucocytes would have been destroyed by an *allograft* reaction (see *adoptive immunity*). Transfer factor is prepared from blood leucocytes that have been disrupted by alternate freezing and thawing, treated by the enzyme deoxyribonuclease and filtered through a *dialysis* membrane.

XENOGRAFT A graft between animals that are distantly related taxonomically, e.g. from a human being to mouse, A transplantation that would be described as 'xenogeneic'.

Y ANTIGENS Transplantation antigens which in some strains of mice differentiate males from females from the same inbred strain and are responsible for the rejection of grafts transplanted from male to female.

Some Common Abbreviations

Ab	antibody
Ag	antigen
BGG	bovine gamma globulin
BSS	balanced salt solution
DLA	dog leucocyte antigen
DNP	2–4 dinitrophenol
EAE	experimental allergic encephalitis
EDTA	ethylene diamine tetracetic acid
FCS	fetal calf serum
HLA	human leucocyte antigen
HSA	human serum albumin
Ig	immunoglobulin
i.p.	intraperitioneal
i.v.	intravenous
KLH	keyhole limpet haemocyanin
MEM	minimal essential medium
MHC	major histocompatibility complex
MLC	mixed leucocyte culture
MLR	mixed leucocyte reaction
NIP	hydroxy-3-iodo-5-nitrophenacetyl
PBS	phosphate buffered saline

s.c.   subcutaneous
TRIS   Trometamol
V   virus
           FSV = Feline sarcoma virus
           MSV = Mouse sarcoma virus
           RSV = Rous sarcoma virus
           TMV = Tobacco mosaic virus

Index

155

Index